A CASEBOOK IN PSYCHIATRIC ETHICS

Report No. 129

A CASEBOOK IN PSYCHIATRIC ETHICS

Formulated by the
Committee on Medical Education

GROUP FOR THE ADVANCEMENT OF PSYCHIATRY

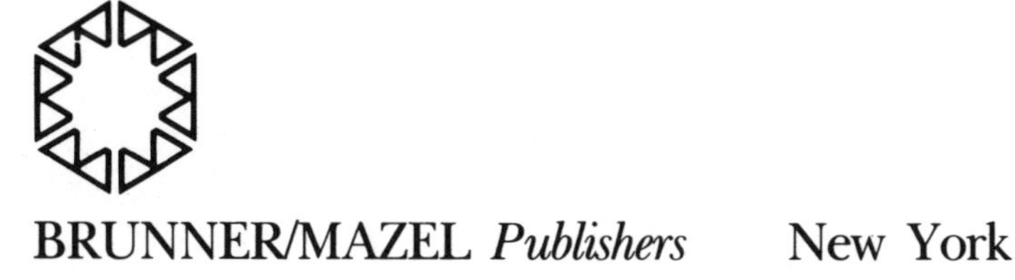

BRUNNER/MAZEL *Publishers* New York

Library of Congress Cataloging-in-Publication Data
A Casebook in psychiatric ethics / formulated by the Committee on Medical Education, Group for the Advancement of Psychiatry.
p. cm. — (Report ; no. 129)
Includes bibliographical references.
ISBN 0-87630-609-1.—ISBN 0-87630-610-5 (pbk.)
1. Psychiatric ethics—Case studies. I. Group for the Advancement of Psychiatry. Committee on Medical Education. II. Series: Report (Group for the Advancement of Psychiatry : 1984) ; no. 129.
[DNLM: 1. Ethics, Medical. 2. Psychiatry. W1 RE209BR no. 129 / WM 62 C3365]
RC321.G7 no. 129
[RC455.2.E8]
616.89 s—dc20
[174'.2]
DNLM/DLC
for Library of Congress 90-2124
CIP

Published by
BRUNNER-MAZEL, INC.
19 Union Square West
New York, New York, 10003

Manufactured in the United States of America

10 9 8 7 6 5 4 3 2 1

STATEMENT OF PURPOSE

THE GROUP FOR THE ADVANCEMENT OF PSYCHIATRY has a membership of approximately 300 psychiatrists, most of whom are organized in the form of a number of working committees. These committees direct their efforts toward the study of various aspects of psychiatry and the application of this knowledge to the fields of mental health and human relations.

Collaboration with specialists in other disciplines has been and is one of GAP's working principles. Since the formation of GAP in 1946, its members have worked closely with such other specialists as anthropologists, biologists, economists, statisticians, educators, lawyers, nurses, psychologists, sociologists, social workers and experts in mass communication, philosophy, and semantics. GAP envisages a continuing program of work according to the following aims:

1. To collect and appraise significant data in the fields of psychiatry, mental health, and human relations;
2. To reevaluate old concepts and to develop and test new ones;
3. To apply the knowledge thus obtained for the promotion of mental health and good human relations.

GAP is an independent group, and its reports represent the composite findings and opinions of its members only, guided by its many consultants.

A Casebook in Psychiatric Ethics was formulated by the Committee on Medical Education. The members of this committee are listed on page vii. The members of the other GAP committees, as well as additional membership categories and current and past officers of GAP, are listed at the end of the report.

Committee on Medical Education
GROUP FOR THE ADVANCEMENT OF PSYCHIATRY

Stephen C. Scheiber, M.D., *Chairman*

Gene M. Abroms, M.D.
Charles M. Culver, M.D., Ph.D.
Steven Dubovsky, M.D.
Saul Harrison, M.D.
David R. Hawkins, M.D.
Harold I. Lief, M.D.
Carol Nadelson, M.D.
Carolyn B. Robinowitz, M.D.
Sidney L. Werkman, M.D.
Veva Zimmerman, M.D.

Bernard Gert, Ph.D., *Consultant*

James Dillon, M.D., *Fellow*
Erol Giray, M.D., *Fellow*
Eric Hollander, M.D., *Fellow*
Kathleen McKenna, M.D., *Fellow*
Mark Sullivan, M.D., Ph.D., *Fellow*

CONTENTS

A CASEBOOK IN PSYCHIATRIC ETHICS

1

INTRODUCTION

Why a Psychiatric Ethics Casebook?

When must a psychiatrist disclose what a patient has said in confidence? Can psychotic patients ever give valid consent to be research subjects? Is it ever ethically justified to overrule the treatment refusal of a competent patient? Is it always inappropriate to have romantic relationships with patients? How about ex-patients? Is the choice of medication versus psychotherapy for a hyperactive child an ethical or an empirical issue?

As these questions suggest, psychiatric practice is filled with ethical* dilemmas and sometimes it is difficult to know whether clinical psychiatric questions are ethical, technical, or both in nature. Psychiatrists often find the ethical decisions they must make in their clinical practice confusing and frustrating. This casebook seeks to clarify this area by examining ethical questions in the context of a series of clinical cases.

One hallmark of a profession is a self-conscious concern with the ethical behavior of its members. In medicine there is evidence of this concern in the earliest recorded medical writings. The Hippocratic Oath, for example, was developed in the 4th century B.C. in Greece; it has some topical interest even today.

---

*In everyday usage the terms "ethical" and "moral" have different connotations for some persons, though many philosophers make no distinction and use them as synonyms. In deference to everyday usage we mostly use "ethical" herein, except in such phrases as "moral philosophy" or "moral rule" which are so entrenched in the field of philosophy that a substitution would be awkward.

However, in recent years, partly in response to the enormous growth of medical technology, public and professional concern with ethical problems in medicine has burgeoned.

A new discipline of biomedical ethics has emerged. The growth of the Hastings Center and the Kennedy Institute at Georgetown University are examples of this expanding field of inquiry. New life-sustaining technologies have raised complex questions about the definition of life itself and about the quality of some lives capable of being prolonged by technology. At the same time medical care has become enormously costly, consuming an ever-increasing percentage of the country's gross national product. Although the de facto rationing of health care is very much with us today, it seems inevitable that further limits on health care consumption will be necessary in the future.

Psychiatry, no less than other specialties, has been a focus of increased ethical concern. While recent developments in psychiatric treatment and case management have not introduced completely novel issues, they have heightened old controversies. Are patients cured or merely controlled by medications that have a profound influence on their behavior and emotions? Are deinstitutionalized patients, many now among the homeless, better off than they were in public mental hospitals? Who should have the authority to decide these questions: the patient, the psychiatrist, the state legislature?

Psychiatrists are increasingly required to be agents of society as well as of the patient. The Tarasoff decision in California, now accepted in many states, established a legal duty for the psychiatrist to take measures to protect an individual who may be in jeopardy from a dangerous patient. This may involve warning the individual, which may require the psychiatrist to violate confidentiality, a duty thought by many to be at the core of the psychiatrist-patient relationship. Is it ethically as well as legally required to breach? The AIDS epidemic raises a similar issue: Should the psychiatrist inform the lover of an HIV+ patient about the patient's seropositivity if the patient does not want him or her to be told?

This casebook is intended to be an introduction to psychiatric ethics. It is directed toward practicing psychiatrists, residents in training, medical students, and other mental health professionals. It is not intended to be a comprehensive textbook although relevant theoretical material has been included in the case discussions. Some of the theoretical material is summarized and expanded upon in the final chapter.

Psychiatry and ethics are two different disciplines, and competence in one does not confer competence in the other (Perl & Shelp, 1982). We believe, however, that if psychiatrists learn some basic concepts in medical ethics, most of them will be competent to manage most of the ethical dilemmas they encounter. Nonetheless there are occasional difficult cases where the help of an outside consultant who has specialized in medical ethics may be valuable. An increasing number of hospitals have established Ethics Advisory Committees, which provide this kind of specialized consultation (Cranford & Doudera, 1984). Many of these committees, in fact, have psychiatrist members. Some psychiatric skills are helpful in performing ethics consultations, and psychiatrists who study medical ethics in depth can become effective ethics consultants.

Ethical Theory

Most cases in this book involve the application of ethical theory to the practice of psychiatry. It is useful for psychiatrists to learn some concepts and theories from medical ethics. Competent psychiatric practice depends on common sense, but common sense is often not enough in and of itself to deal with difficult ethical dilemmas.

Many books in applied ethics begin with one or more chapters summarizing ethical theory and then proceed to professional applications. We have chosen a different approach. We use cases from the outset, but put them in a sequence, especially in the first parts of the book, so that ethical concepts and theory are gradually introduced.

There is no one ethical theory that is universally accepted. A diversity of ethical theories can, in fact, be described and their names and subdivisions can be daunting to the newcomer: subjectivism; emotivism; act- and rule-utilitarianism; deontology; and the like. We try to provide here the framework of an understandable general ethical theory which can be usefully applied to important issues in psychiatry. The theorist to whom we are most indebted is Bernard Gert (1989). Gert's "contractarianism" approach, like that of Rawls (1971), combines many features of utilitarianism (Mill, 1863) and deontology (Kant, 1785; Ross, 1930).

The American Medical Association's *Principles of Medical Ethics*

In this Casebook frequent reference will be found to the AMA's *Principles of Medical Ethics,* especially to the annotated version published by the American Psychiatric Association (1986). The relevant parts of this booklet may be seen in the Appendix of this Casebook. This APA booklet, and the associated *Opinion of the Ethics Committee on the Principles of Medical Ethics* booklet (1985) should be familiar to every psychiatric resident and practicing psychiatrist. A great deal of thought has gone into the formulation of these annotations and opinions, and they cover many important topics and situations in professional practice.

This Casebook complements the two APA booklets, but it has a somewhat different emphasis. The AMA's *Principles* and the APA's *Annotations* and *Opinions* focus on the kinds of conduct and kinds of professional practice that the booklets label as ethical or unethical. There is less attention to underlying ethical theory and concepts, which is appropriate because that is not the purpose of the booklets. For example, although the *Annotations* volume mentions the concept of "informed consent" it nowhere focuses on it explicitly or gives a definition of valid consent and refusal. On the other hand, the APA booklets cover a far greater number of professional situations than a book like this could hope to address.

Ethics and Law

Although this Casebook occasionally touches on matters of health law, the discussion is devoted largely to ethics. There is health law, both case and statutory, which is germane to many of the cases presented here, and it is useful for psychiatrists to know that law. For example, different states have different legal standards for specifying the nature of a physician's duty to disclose information during the consent process; many states, especially in the courts, have confronted the issue of when treatment may and may not be given to unwilling patients; and having sexual relations with patients exposes a psychiatrist to legal liability as well as to ethical censure.

We have not discussed health law in detail for several reasons. One is simply lack of space. Another is that we believe health law is best taught through a systematic presentation of its own, and not as ancillary to ethics or some other subject. Issues of negligent professional practice, for example, are best understood after appreciating in detail the nature of personal injury liability, and such matters would have taken us too far afield.

We also believe it is important for psychiatrists to be able to conceptualize ethical issues clearly, holding the relevant law temporarily in abeyance. In that way they can avoid the temptation of trying to decide what is ethical by trying to decide what is "legal." Law and ethics are related but they are not the same thing. Also, there often is no "law" which clearly applies to a specific psychiatric dilemma.

It is almost always true that if psychiatrists have sound ethical reasons for a course of action, discuss them with a colleague if at all unsure how to proceed, and clearly document their thinking in the patient's chart, they need not worry overmuch that they have broken some law or exposed themselves needlessly to a charge of liability.

The Casebook Format

The casebook format was chosen because we believe that the case method is at the heart of medical education. Moral rules and conflicts arise frequently in individual clinical cases and can be effectively studied initially in that context. The seventeen cases presented here represent actual problems encountered in the experience of the members of the Committee on Medical Education. The cases have been altered slightly in the interest of confidentiality. All of the names used are fictitious.

The seventeen cases have been grouped into five chapters. The first chapter is that of *valid consent and refusal.* Many important ethical problems in psychiatry are related to the duty that psychiatrists have to try to obtain a valid consent or refusal, and what they are ethically allowed or required to do in the event that a valid consent or refusal cannot be obtained. The second chapter deals with *problems in psychiatric paternalism.* Psychiatrists are often confronted with the dilemma of whether it is ethically justified to act paternalistically, for example, to hospitalize someone who does not want to enter a hospital, or to medicate someone who refuses medication.

The third chapter presents three cases of ethical problems that can arise in *relationships with colleagues:* a resident who believes his supervisor's directives are not in a patient's best interest; a resident who believes a supervisor has become impaired in his clinical functioning; and a community mental health center psychiatrist who signs blank prescription forms which will later be completed by nonmedical colleagues. A fourth chapter contains two cases involving *romantic or sexual attraction between psychiatrists and patients.* A fifth chapter presents three cases, two concerning the breaching of *confidentiality,* and one concerning certain *double-agentry* problems raised by many of the new financial arrangements for reimbursing psychiatric care.

Each case begins with a case history, followed by a discussion section, which introduces relevant ethical concepts and theory. Each discussion section ends with one or more questions designed to probe more widely or deeply into the issues raised by that case.

The discussion sections provide some useful conceptualizations of the issues raised in each case. Often we suggest what we believe are ethically appropriate ways for the psychiatrist to proceed. We do not intend to be dogmatic. Moral philosophy is not a univocal discipline and there are alternative ways to conceptualize the issues underlying some of the cases. It is also true that reasonable persons might disagree with some of the recommendations we make about how cases should be resolved. Exploring and debating these differences would be a useful teaching activity. We have tried hard to be clear in our exposition and our arguments so that those who disagree may at least be able to locate readily the source of their disagreement.

Some but not all discussion sections assume a familiarity with previously discussed material. Thus cases 1-5 should precede cases 6-9 and the cases within these two chapters should mostly be read in order. Cases in the last three chapters can be read in any order, and do not depend greatly on the first two chapters, though there are occasional allusions to earlier material. A few pertinent references are included at the end of the chapters, though these are not exhaustive bibliographies.

We have selected cases that, while not simple, usually raise one issue at a time. Real cases often raise more than one issue simultaneously, and issues can be nested within issues in complex ways. However this simpler treatment seemed more appropriate for an introductory casebook. While the issues discussed here are important issues in psychiatric ethics, we make no claim for having raised all of the important issues in the field.

Using the Casebook in Teaching

Although the Casebook can simply be read as a text, we believe the better teaching method is small-group discussion. There are several ways a small group can work with this material. One that we have used with residents is to confine the early part of the group's discussion to an analysis of the factual part of the case, even though everyone may have read the entire case before the meeting: What issues does the case raise? What additional information, if any, might it be useful for the psychiatrist to obtain before proceeding? What would be the advantages and disadvantages of various ways in which the psychiatrist could act? It may be helpful for the group leader to play a neutral but active facilitating role at this point, perhaps listing relevant issues and concepts on a blackboard as the group teases them out. After a period of free-ranging discussion to the factual circumstances of the case, the group might turn to our discussion section, evaluate its usefulness, and perhaps suggest additional or alternative formulations to ours.

The questions at the end of the discussion sections should be valuable for most groups to address. Some questions are more difficult than others but the discussion of any of them should deepen the reader's appreciation of the subject at hand.

We hope that this casebook will help psychiatrists see that all cases have important ethical dimensions. Much of the time these dimensions are not obvious because the psychiatrist involved acts in an ethically appropriate and uncontroversial manner. The ethical dimensions of a case become more conspicuous when the psychiatrist faces conflicting ethical duties. Our goal has been to increase the reader's ability to recognize and describe ethical dilemmas, to isolate the conflicting duties they contain, and to try to achieve an ethically appropriate resolution. We hope the casebook will sensitize psychiatrists to their diverse ethical responsibilities toward patients, patients' families, and colleagues, and thereby improve the care of all patients.

We want to express our gratitude to the many psychiatrists, psychiatric residency training directors, and house officers who have critiqued earlier versions of the Casebook. They have added considerably to its scope and clarity.

References

American Psychiatric Association. (1985). *Opinion of the Ethics Committee on the Principles of Medical Ethics.* Washington, DC: APA.

American Psychiatric Association. (1986). *The principles of medical ethics with annotations especially applicable to psychiatry.* Washington, DC: APA.

Cranford, R. E., & Doudera, A. E. (1984). *Institutional ethics committees and health care decision making*. Ann Arbor: Health Administration Press.
Gert, B. (1989). *Morality*. New York: Oxford.
Kant, I. (1785). *Groundwork of the metaphysics of morals.*
Mill, J. S. (1863). *Utilitarianism.*
Perl, M., and Shelp, E. E. (1982). Psychiatric consultation masking moral dilemmas in medicine. *New England Journal of Medicine, 307*, 618–620.
Rawls, J. (1971). *A theory of justice.* Cambridge, MA: Harvard University Press.
Ross, D. (1930). *The right and the good.* New York: Oxford.

2
VALID CONSENT AND REFUSAL

CASE 1. THE CRITERIA FOR VALID CONSENT AND REFUSAL

Mrs. Arnold, a 35-year-old married woman, was seen by Dr. Monarda at the request of her internist. She had been troubled in recent years by symptoms of anxiety which, over the past several months, had been taking the form of frequent discrete panic attacks, recently occurring almost every day. She had begun to avoid driving her car, fearing that an attack might occur while she was in the middle of heavy traffic. Her internist had found her to be in excellent physical health and could find no physical cause for her anxiety symptoms.

Dr. Monarda conducted a psychiatric examination and concluded that Mrs. Arnold was suffering from a Panic Disorder. He assured her that there are several treatments available for her problem, that the vast majority of patients, 80–90% or more, can be helped significantly, and that perhaps half of that number can become essentially symptom-free. Without treatment, her symptoms would be likely to continue or even worsen for the indefinite future, though there was some chance (25–30%?) that they might lessen or disappear on their own.

Dr. Monarda recommended a trial of short-term psychotherapy, combined with tricyclic antidepressant (TCA) medication. He told Mrs. Arnold that while there were no completely satisfactory statistics available, he believed that this combination of treatments offered the best chance of success. He did tell her, however, that some practitioners use behavioral therapy or psychotherapy alone for her condition and others use medication alone, and that in fact there is more than one kind of drug that may be used.

Mrs. Arnold agreed to Dr. Monarda's suggested plan but asked to be told more about the medication part of it. He explained that TCAs, often in a lower dose than that used to treat depression, are frequently useful in either preventing or reducing the severity of panic attacks. He mentioned that there are other types of medication that are also sometimes successful, but that TCAs require no dietary restrictions and that tolerance to them rarely develops, as is the case with some of the other kinds of drugs. She asked if there were any drawbacks to taking TCAs. Dr. Monarda described the frequently encountered but nonserious anticholinergic side effects. Since she had no history of glaucoma or of any cardiac problems, he told her that a TCA would be a safe drug for her to take. He explained that while serious reactions to TCAs are seen on rare occasions, as is true of nearly every drug prescribed or sold over the counter, they are almost unknown, and in her case would be on the order of 1 in 10,000 or less.

Mrs. Arnold agreed to proceed with the treatment plan. Dr. Monarda saw her weekly for three months; on three occasions her husband accompanied her. She was given a prescription for imipramine, 50 mg, HS, which she took for six months. Her panic attacks lessened in frequency and duration after the first two or three weeks of treatment and had essentially disappeared after three months. When last heard from, six months after discontinuing the medication, she remained symptom-free.

Discussion

On the face of it, this case might seem to have little to do with medical ethics. Yet the interaction between Dr. Monarda and Mrs. Arnold can be described using rich and important philosophical concepts.

One of the most important ethical questions to ask about any clinical transaction is whether the consent or refusal obtained from the patient is valid. There are three requirements for a valid consent or refusal:

1) The information given to the patient must be adequate.
2) No coercion may have been used in obtaining the consent.
3) The patient must be fully competent to consent or refuse.

The three criteria for a valid consent were satisfied or reasonably well satisfied in this case. Thus the case is relatively unproblematic from an ethical point of view. But it is useful to be aware of the various ethical features that are contained in essentially all clinical transactions in order to be better prepared to analyze those cases that are ethically problematic. The three criteria for a valid consent or refusal will be briefly explained here; a more extended discussion is in the final chapter.

Adequate Information. Patients must receive adequate information about any tests, procedures or treatments proposed to them. The general rule is that any information should be given that a rational person would want to know before making a decision. The minimum that a rational person would want to know is the likely harms and benefits associated with the suggested treatment, with any reasonable alternative treatment(s), and with no treatment at all.

In the above example, Mrs. Arnold appears to have been given a fairly thorough account of the harms and benefits associated with the treatment alternatives open to her. Can you think of anything she was not told about treatment that a rational person might want to know?

No Coercion. Coercion involves the use of such powerful negative incentives, for example, threats of severe pain or significant deprivation of freedom, that it would be unreasonable to expect a patient to resist them. The use of coercion is sometimes morally justified, but any resultant "consent" by the patient is not valid. Psychiatrists are frequently coercive when they threaten patients with commitment to state hospitals if the patients do not continue their "voluntary" treatment elsewhere. Attempts to influence that apply milder degrees of pressure are not coercive. There is no indication at all that Mrs. Arnold was coerced into consenting.

Patient Competence. A patient is competent to consent to or refuse treatment when she understands and appreciates the information given to her during the consent process. A patient understands information if she adequately comprehends the meaning of what she has been told; she appreciates the information if she realizes that what she has been told does indeed apply to her at the present time. Competence thus refers to a patient's cognitive abilities to process information; it does not refer to whether a patient has or has not consented to treatment. Mrs. Arnold appears to be fully competent: she apparently understood and appreciated the information given to her by Dr. Monarda.

Discussion Questions

1. What are three ways in which the case could be altered to show a patient consent which was invalid because of not satisfying, respectively, the three necessary criteria?
2. Can you think of instances from your own experience in which the consent given by psychiatric patients has been invalid according to the above three criteria? Do you think the validity of consent varies significantly in different clinical settings? When it is invalid, which of the three criteria is most frequently unsatisfied?
3. Think of a patient with whom you have recently begun some form of psychodynamic psychotherapy. According to the above criteria, what would constitute an adequate disclosure of information to the patient about the possible harms and benefits of the treatment process?

References

Beauchamp, T. L., & Childress, J. F. (1989). *Principles of biomedical ethics* (3rd ed. pp. 74–111). New York: Oxford.

Culver, C. M., & Gert, B. (1982). *Philosophy in medicine* (pp. 42–63). New York: Oxford.

Katz, J. (1984). *The silent world of doctor and patient,* New York: Free Press.

CASE 2. FAMILY COERCION AND VALID CONSENT

It was noted in Case 1 that coercion by the physician invalidates a patient's consent. But what if the coercion comes not from the physician but from a member of the patient's family?

Mrs. Pinfold was a 61-year-old, legally blind woman who was transferred to a psychiatric inpatient unit from a nearby community hospital for treatment of a recurrent depression. She had had three episodes of depression over the past 10 years, each of which had responded poorly to drug treatment but subsequently was resolved with ECT. She suffered from marked atherosclerosis and three years previously had experienced a moderately severe myocardial infarction.

Review of her recent history and present medications, plus physical and mental status examinations, added no further information to suggest that her current depressive symptomatology was due to anything other than recurrent unipolar depression. Her symptoms on admission included a decreased appetite, mid-cycle and early morning awakening, diurnal mood variation, anhedonia, and lack of energy. However, she had maintained adequate food and fluid intake and had lost no weight. There was no evidence of any psychotic thought process, and she denied suicidal or homicidal ideation. Thus, while it seemed she would be helped by ECT, there appeared to be no strong moral or legal justification for forcing it upon her. Over the past three months adequate doses of three different kinds of antidepressant drugs had been given, with Mrs. Pinfold's valid consent, but none had had significant effect.

She came to the inpatient unit following a consulting psychiatrist's recommendation that she receive ECT for her depression. A cardiology consultant felt that there was no medical contraindication to ECT and that, in fact, because of her cardiac history, ECT would be safer than increased doses of antidepressant medication. At the time of transfer, Mrs. Pinfold had agreed with the plans for ECT.

However, two days after admission, when her psychiatrist, Dr. Cohen, approached her to discuss ECT, she told Dr. Cohen that she was afraid to have ECT and would consent only because her husband was putting great pressure on her to do so. She wanted help with her depression but, despite the cardiologist's reassurance, she was frightened that ECT would cause another heart attack. She said that her husband had threatened her at the time of admission by saying he would not help care for her at home if she returned without having had ECT. Because of her blindness and her cardiac condition, she required much assistance at home with personal hygiene and with dressing and feeding herself. She had no close friends or relatives whom she could ask for assistance at home. Although numerous attempts by various health care workers to contact Mr. Pinfold over the next week proved unsuccessful, he did tell his wife by telephone that he would refuse to come to the hospital or talk to any staff member until she had had ECT. Mrs. Pinfold asked the staff to stop trying to reach her husband. She said that she was willing to give permission for ECT, and sign a consent form, though she continued to tell the staff that if it were up to her alone, she would not consent.

Discussion

The treatment staff was unsure what to do. Mrs. Pinfold clearly regarded it as impossible to return home without her husband's support. There was no one else with whom she could stay. Discharging her to a state-supported nursing home might be possible, but the psychiatric care there would be substandard and she, herself, rejected this notion. Under the circumstances, Mr. Pinfold's behavior represented coercion: He was threatening his wife with such a powerful negative incentive—the loss of the only adequate home environment available to her—that it would be unreasonable to expect her to be able to refuse his attempt to control her.

Two of the criteria for establishing the validity of her consent were clearly met: she had been given adequate information about ECT, and she seemed to understand and appreciate this information. Did her husband's coercion invalidate the consent she was prepared to give?

We believe her consent should be regarded as valid. The physicians were not coercing her, and they had no control over the coercing party. Her husband's coercion was simply a fact-about-her-life with which she had to contend, much as someone suffering from appendicitis must contend with her abdominal pain in deciding whether to consent to an appendectomy. In each case, the patient's decision is determined by a strong negative stimulus for which the physician bears no responsibility and over which the physician has no control. While Mr. Pinfold's paternalistic behavior toward his wife was probably ethically unjustified (see below for a discussion of paternalistic behavior and its justification), the doctors did not have Mrs. Pinfold's consent to intervene with her husband. Her consent was valid, and her physicians were ethically justified in proceeding with ECT treatment. Refusal to treat would bring about the paradoxical situation of withholding the one treatment that seemed medically indicated and that had been requested by the patient.

Discussion Questions

1. Suppose Mrs. Pinfold asked you to intervene and convince her husband not to insist upon ECT. What, if anything, would you feel ethically justified in doing?

2. Suppose the case were changed in the following way: Dr. Cohen, as above, believes Mrs. Pinfold should have ECT but is unable to persuade her to do so. Mr. Pinfold also believes his wife should have ECT but has played no active role in trying to change her mind. Dr. Cohen knows that Mr. Pinfold is a forceful person, and that his wife depends a great deal upon him. Dr. Cohen convinces Mr. Pinfold that it would be so much in his wife's best interests to have ECT that he should coerce her into doing so. Mr. Pinfold successfully coerces her, as above, and Mrs. Pinfold reluctantly consents. Was Mrs. Pinfold's consent valid? Was it ethically justified for her physicians to arrange for her to be coerced by her husband?

Reference

Mallary, S. D., Gert, B., & Culver, C. M. (1986). Family coercion and valid consent. *Theoretical Medicine, 7,* 123–126.

CASE 3. COMPETENCE TO CONSENT OR REFUSE

Mr. Jones is a 67-year-old retired farmer who lives alone and has no close relatives. Two years ago he had a skin lesion, which proved to be a malignant melanoma, and was treated with surgery and chemotherapy. However, his cancer has recently recurred and is now more widespread than before. At the time of his current admission he is judged to be terminally ill. His physicians are recommending further debulking surgery and another course of chemotherapy, feeling these procedures may afford him appreciable relief from pain and possibly extend his life by a few months. Mr. Jones has declined these treatments, however, and says that he simply wants to go home and await his death. He has been seen by a psychiatric consultant who feels he is not clinically depressed.

Except in very rare cases, there is no moral or legal justification for overruling the treatment refusal of a competent patient. But is Mr. Jones competent? The treating staff feels some uncertainty about this issue. During the past year he has had two strokes, which have left him with some mild but definite cognitive impairment. He cannot perform mental calculations nearly as well as he once could, and his recent memory is somewhat impaired. However, he seems to understand his medical situation adequately. He knows the facts about the nature of his illness and about the probable course of his illness with and without further treatment.

Mr. Jones's physicians do not feel strongly impelled to attempt to force treatment upon him, or even to pressure him very strongly to have it. The dilemma they feel, and which they present to the psychiatric consultant, is whether it is justified to regard Mr. Jones as competent to refuse treatment. Can a cognitively impaired man be competent?

Discussion

It is important for psychiatrists to understand clearly the concept of competence, since they are frequently asked by their medical and surgical colleagues to assess that ability in patients. The courts also frequently request a psychiatrist's opinion about a patient's competence to consent to or refuse treatment.

One frequent source of confusion about competence is that patients are often, in a shorthand fashion, referred to as simply competent or incompetent. However, competence is best understood not as a global characteristic, so that patients are either wholly competent or wholly incompetent, but rather as a collection of abilities, so that persons may be competent to do some things but not competent to do others. For example, a patient may be competent to feed himself, but incompetent to consent to or refuse treatment. While there are some persons who are not competent to do anything, for example, the comatose, there is no one who is competent to do everything, so in assessing a noncomatose patient's competence, it is always necessary to ask: Competent to do what? Criteria can then be used which must be satisfied in order to be judged competent to do that particular thing.

It was suggested above that competence to consent to or refuse treatment is best understood as a patient's ability to understand and appreciate the information conveyed during the consent process. Mr. Jones did understand and appreciate this information, so he should be judged competent to consent to or refuse further treatment. He may be, by contrast, no longer competent to do serial sevens or to recall a set of memorized objects after a five-minute interval. These incompetencies, however, do not affect the fact that he adequately understands and appreciates the information pertinent to his medical situation, and he should therefore be classified as competent to consent or refuse.

The definition of competence used here is widely accepted and is consonant with many states' statutory definition of competence and also with some states' case law. There is, nonetheless, some theoretical dispute about whether the concept of competence is best defined in this way. Some writers wish, in one way or another, to incorporate into the concept not only the patient's understanding and appreciation of information, but also the rationality of the decision that the patient actually makes. We believe the concepts of one's competence to consent or refuse, and the rationality of that decision once it is made, are best kept conceptually separate. We will explain this theoretical dispute about the definition of competence in more detail in the final chapter. The concept of rationality will be explained in Case 6.

Discussion Question

1. Suppose the case were altered so that the clinical facts were the same but Mr. Jones was no longer fully competent to refuse. For example, suppose he consistently refused the surgery and said he wanted to go home and die, but did not seem to understand that the surgery would likely give him a significant degree of pain relief. Would it follow directly from his compromised competence that it was justified to treat him over his objections? What does that imply about the importance of a patient's competence in making decisions about whether to overrule his refusal of treatment?

References

Beauchamp, T. L., & Childress, J. F. (1989). *Principles of biomedical ethics*, 3rd Ed. New York: Oxford, 79–85.

Culver, C. M. (1986). The clinical determination of competence. In M. B. Kapp, H. E. Pies, & A. E. Doudera (Eds.), *Legal and ethical aspects of health care for the elderly* (pp. 277–285). Ann Arbor, MI: Health Administration Press.

Culver, C. M., & Gert, B. (1982). *Philosophy in medicine* (pp. 52–62). New York: Oxford.

CASE 4. THE CONSENT TO OR REFUSAL OF TREATMENT BY CHILDREN

Eric was an eight-year-old child who was referred to Dr. Kim because of his maladaptive behavior in school. Throughout his schooling, Eric had required more supervision than his peers because of his disruptiveness, his difficulty in awaiting his turn, and his inability to remain seated and sustain attention on a task. Although his academic performance was average, this was much below his potential as measured by a variety of intellectual tests. His parents had always perceived Eric as more "energetic" than his siblings. The information supplied by the parents and by Eric's teacher verbally, and supported by elevations in Conners Hyperactivity Scale scores, was quite consistent with the diagnosis of Attention-Deficit Hyperactivity Disorder (ADHD).

Family sessions conveyed the impression of a warm, well-structured family headed by two loving, sensitive, supportive parents who employed appropriate reinforcements in response to Eric's "exuberant" behavior, as they designated it. It also seemed that Eric's sister Kate, who was two years older, did not gain any inappropriate advantages as a consequence of Eric's problems.

On the basis of individual sessions with Eric, Dr. Kim hypothesized that intrapsychic conflicts might also play some role in his disorder. Eric typically inhibited the expression of aggression. For example, more than once while playing checkers, Eric became fidgety and tense and stared for extended periods at an obvious jump he could make of one of Dr. Kim's checkers and then, failing to take the jump, moved his piece in some other direction. When Dr. Kim asked Eric why he had decided not to jump, Eric responded loudly and excitedly in a manner that suggested he was afraid of retaliation.

Dr. Kim knew that anxiety is considered by many to be the most frequent cause of hyperactivity in children. An intrapsychic conflict about aggression could be a cause of anxiety and, in a patient of Eric's age, the anxiety could very well be expressed through motor activity. But Dr. Kim was also aware that since Eric had suffered from hyperactivity since very early childhood, his conflicts about aggression and self-esteem might well reflect psychological reactions to an underlying ADHD.

Contact with Eric's school confirmed the parents' report.

The teacher said Eric had difficulty staying with a task, and described him as often too aggressive, though usually remorseful after the fact. Despite his frequent difficulties with peers, he maintained school friendships similar to his parents' description of his adjustment in the neighborhood.

Dr. Kim perceived no signs of family dysfunction prominent enough to suggest that family therapy was indicated. He thought also that the parents had intuitively modeled and instructed Eric in cognitive mediations of behavior, almost as if they had read and applied techniques from the burgeoning cognitive behavioral literature on ADHD. Further, the behavioral reinforcement offered by the schools and parents seemed close to optimal.

Dr. Kim therefore felt there were two principal treatment options: 1) individual psychotherapy, and 2) pharmacotherapy with a stimulant medication. Each had important potential harms and benefits. Psychotherapy might be useful in helping Eric with his apparent intrapsychic conflicts about aggression by uncovering sources other than his presumptive ADHD. In addition, both the patient and his parents seemed eager to engage in psychotherapy.

On the other hand, psychotherapy might be of limited value in successfully resolving specific ADHD symptoms, if intrapsychic conflicts were not the basis of Eric's hyperactivity symptoms. Pharmacotherapy, on the other hand, might lead to a rapid and inexpensive reduction in symptoms and, if it were not effective in a timely manner, psychotherapy could then be instituted. Drug therapy, however, carried some risk of side effects. Dr. Kim concluded that either or both treatment options could be followed reasonably, so he advised that the decision should be made by the family.

In Eric's presence, Dr. Kim described to the parents the potential benefits and harms associated with the two treatments. The parents asked Dr. Kim's opinion. He replied that he thought it would be simplest and most economical to start with a trial of stimulant medication coupled with further evaluation of Eric, ongoing consultation with the family, and the use of serial Conners scales by Eric's teacher. Psychotherapy could then be employed if medication did not prove to be helpful. The parents agreed with this course of action. Eric, however, strongly objected. He said he was willing to continue to talk with Dr. Kim, but also said he did not want to take any medicine and did not want his teacher to be asked to fill out scales about him. Eric seemed to understand reasonably well what Dr. Kim had said about each of the treatment alternatives. Was he competent to refuse? Does that matter? Should his refusal be respected?

Discussion

The subject of children's "competence" to consent to or refuse treatment is complex. It is commonly said, and the law sometimes seems to parallel this kind of thinking, that children are "incompetent" to make treatment decisions, and that parents should therefore be relied upon to make proxy decisions for their children. But it seems clear that many persons under the age of 18 are fully competent to make decisions, if "competence" is defined as the ability to understand and appreciate the information given during the consent process. If competence is defined in this way then very young children, roughly age 6 and below, would usually not be fully competent to decide; older children, roughly age 13 to 17, usually would be competent to decide; those in between, like Eric, roughly age 8 to 11, might be competent to understand and appreciate the information given for some simple treatment decisions, but not for a decision with any sort of complexity of information. In this case, Eric did seem competent to understand and appreciate the information that Dr. Kim had given.*

However, the concept of "competence" is not sufficient to account for our moral intuitions about the weight that should be given to children's consents or refusals. Most physicians feel that parents should be given nearly total authority over medical

*The recent GAP report, *How Old is Old Enough* (1989), contains a scholarly exploration of these developmental issues related to consent by children.

and other decisions concerning children until about the age of 12, so long as the parents' decision is a rational one. This is true even if a child like Eric does understand and appreciate the information about the treatment(s) being suggested. One important reason for not allowing young children to make treatment decisions is that they are frequently incapable of adequately weighing short-term against long-term harms and benefits. They may refuse a treatment to avoid some immediate but short-term pain or discomfort, even though they may thereby be incurring the risk of much more serious suffering at some future time. Eric appeared to be making a decision on this basis. As children become older, especially when they reach the mid-teen years of 15 to 17, their decisions should be and are given much more weight and in some instances their parents are not allowed to overrule them. There are, as yet, no well worked-out guidelines for deciding disputes about medical treatment that arise between mid-teenagers and their parents. It is an area that could profit from systematic study.

Eric's parents insisted that he take methylphenidate, and he complied. Dr. Kim accordingly prescribed the drug. Dr. Kim, in turn, complied with Eric's wishes that his teachers not fill out rating scales, and no ratings were done. After two months of drug therapy, Eric's behavior noticeably stabilized. He became more comfortable expressing aggression, and less impulsive and hyperactive. His academic performance, however, did not improve commensurately, so individual academic tutoring with a psychologically sophisticated tutor was instituted. Eric was pleased and his parents continued to consent throughout to the tutoring.

Discussion Questions

1. Do you believe Eric's parents were ethically justified in insisting that he take medication? If not, should Dr. Kim have prescribed it?

2. What guidelines would you suggest for resolving the uncommon but troublesome disputes that arise when a 15–17-

year-old adolescent disagrees with his or her parents about whether a suggested treatment be accepted? Does it make a difference if the adolescent consents and the parents refuse, or if the parents consent and the adolescent refuses? What relative weightings should be assigned to the gravity of the illness and the potential benefit of the treatment?

References

Group for the Advancement of Psychiatry. (1989). *How old is old enough? The ages of rights and responsibilities.* New York: Brunner/Mazel.
Holder, A. (1987). Minors' rights to consent to medical care. *Journal of the American Medical Association, 257,* 3400–3402.

CASE 5. CONSENTING TO RESEARCH

Dr. Gath is a third-year resident at a psychiatric research unit. It is her responsibility to ask for consent to enter a research protocol from Mr. Davis, a 27-year-old man who is an inpatient on the unit. In the past the patient has suffered from several acute psychotic episodes, which have been reliably diagnosed as schizophrenia, paranoid type. He is currently in a remitted state, about to be discharged, with no hallucinations or delusions and only mild residual symptoms. The anticipated research studies include a CT scan of his brain, a lumbar puncture, intravenous blood drawing, and two experimental drugs to be given serially but intermixed with placebo trials. The purpose of the study is to examine the effects of the drugs on certain neurotransmitters. What should Dr. Gath tell Mr. Davis during the consent process?

Discussion

The ethical principles governing the obtaining of consent to research are not different in kind from those for obtaining consent to treatment: Patients need to be given full information, their consent cannot be coerced, and they must be fully competent to consent. It is especially the case that in research that holds no benefit for the patient, the scope of information disclosure should be unusually thorough.

In nearly all institutions that conduct research on human subjects, the research protocol must be approved by an in-house Institutional Review Board (IRB). IRBs critique many aspects of research protocols. They focus specifically on the consent process: Is the scope of disclosure adequately broad? Will information be imparted in language subjects can understand? Do the subjects know that they can withdraw their consent at any time, even after the research has begun? (See Levine, 1986, for an excellent review of ethical issues and regulatory policy in human experimentation.)

Dr. Gath, in talking with Mr. Davis, emphasized especially that the research procedures were not treatments, and that while they might contribute valuable information toward useful future treatments, they would almost certainly not be directly beneficial to him. Each procedure was described in detail, along with its possible negative side effects or complications. Mr. Davis was told that although he was being asked to consent, he could refuse to enter the experiment without any penalty. Dr. Gath also emphasized that, if Mr. Davis did consent, he could withdraw his consent at any time during the research process. Thus, Dr. Gath tried to apply as little pressure as possible in asking for Mr. Davis's consent. Finally, Dr. Gath tested Mr. Davis's understanding and appreciation of the information he had been given in order to insure that Mr. Davis was fully competent to consent to the protocol.

Mr. Davis did consent and participated in the research without any significant adverse side effects. Although Mr. Davis was not psychotic at the time his consent was obtained, the presence of psychotic symptoms would not have barred his giving a valid consent; the critical issue would be whether the symptoms interfered with his ability to understand and appreciate the relevant information. It would be especially important that he thoroughly understand any risks involved and the fact that the procedures would not benefit him in any way.

Discussion Questions

1. Suppose someone argued that adult psychiatric patients are similar to 10-year-old children: that even if they are competent to consent (i.e., they do understand and appreciate the information given to them about the research), they should not be allowed to consent to nontherapeutic research that carries more than trivial risks. (Some people take that position with respect to nontherapeutic research with children.) How would you respond?

2. Suppose that Dr. Gath believed, on the basis of her interview, that Mr. Davis actually did not want to participate but was agreeing to do so to please her. How would you advise her to proceed?

Reference

Levine, R. J. (1986). *Ethics and regulation of clinical research* (2nd ed.). Baltimore: Urban & Schwarzenberg.

3
PATERNALISM IN PSYCHIATRY

CASE 6. TREATING UNWILLING PATIENTS: FIRST CASE

Mr. Brody, a 58-year-old man, was admitted to a psychiatric inpatient unit because of a major depressive episode. He did not wish to be admitted but did not physically resist. Several antidepressant medications had been given to him before admission; none had been very helpful, and he recently had refused to take any medication. He stated that he wanted to die and he refused all food and fluids, hoping to starve to death. The treating psychiatrist, Dr. Lynn, believed he should be given ECT, but Mr. Brody refused. He had no delusions and seemed to understand his situation quite well. He knew his doctors believed he had a probably reversible illness and that they also believed that ECT would be an effective treatment. He also understood quite well that his refusal of food and fluids would eventually lead to his death. He stated that he once enjoyed life but was now so depressed that he did not want to be "cured" and wished to die.

His wife and children believed he should have ECT and, at Dr. Lynn's suggestion, began the process of attempting to obtain guardianship through a probate court. Mrs. Brody wanted to obtain sufficient legal guardianship power to enable her to make medical decisions for her husband, even if they went against his wishes. In the meantime the patient became weaker and weaker, and the treatment team feared that his worsening state of dehydration might precipitate a cardiac dysrhythmia (he had a history of heart disease). Dr. Lynn believed it would be prudent to administer IV fluids while awaiting the probate court decision. Mr. Brody, however, refused to give permission for an IV line to be inserted. What should Dr. Lynn do?

Discussion

This case raises a number of issues in psychiatric ethics: Was Mr. Brody competent to refuse? Was his refusal rational or irrational? Would it be morally justified to treat him (start an IV line) in the face of his refusal? To answer these questions we must define several additional concepts and describe an important decision-making procedure in medical ethics: When is it morally justified to act paternalistically toward a patient?

The Definition of Paternalistic Behavior. The treatment of an unwilling patient almost always represents an example of paternalistic behavior. One useful way to define paternalistic behavior* is to say that behavior is paternalistic when it satisfies four criteria:

1) it is carried out with the intention of benefiting the subject (the patient, in this context);
2) it involves the violation of a moral rule with respect to the patient (see below);
3) it is carried out without the consent of the patient;
4) the patient is at least partially competent or is expected to become at least partially competent in the future.

The only element of this definition we have not yet discussed is "the violation of a moral rule." Violating a moral rule involves acting toward someone in a way that either directly inflicts a harm (by which we mean death, pain, disability, or loss of freedom or pleasure), or increases the likelihood that the person will suffer one or more harms (for example, deceiving

---

*See the final chapter for a more extended discussion of the definition of paternalism.

someone or breaking a promise). Violating a moral rule with respect to someone is always unethical if one does not have an adequate justification for doing so.

In the above case, inserting an IV line would clearly be paternalistic: It would be done with the intention of benefiting the patient; it would violate the moral rules against causing pain and depriving of freedom; it would be done without the patient's consent; and the patient was (at least partially) competent to refuse.

The Ethical Justification of Paternalistic Behavior. Sometimes the paternalistic treatment of unwilling patients is ethically justified and sometimes it is not. In order for it to be ethically justified to treat against a patient's wishes, several ethically relevant criteria must all be satisfied:

1) The harm or harms the treatment will probably avoid or ameliorate for the patient must be very great (for example, death or serious permanent disability).
2) The harm or harms imposed by the treatment must be, by comparison, very much less.
3) The patient's desire not to be treated must be seriously irrational.
4) The above three criteria all refer to characteristics of the particular case under consideration. It is necessary that they be satisfied to justify forced treatment, but it is not sufficient. It must also be the case that rational persons would advocate always allowing forced treatment in cases having the same morally relevant characteristics described by the first three criteria. This fourth criterion forces the kind of impartiality which is a necessary component of ethical reasoning.

The Definition of Irrationality. This decision-making procedure requires that, among other things, a patient's treatment refusal must be seriously irrational. What is an irrational decision or action? A simple but not very precise way of defining an irrational decision or action (and some treatment decisions are irrational decisions) is that it involves hurting oneself pointlessly, as in "cutting off one's nose to spite one's face."

It is useful to express this same idea in more precise language. We will say *a decision or action is irrational if its foreseeable results are that the person will suffer harms without an adequate reason.* We have defined harms; what is an adequate reason?

A *reason* is a conscious belief that one's decision or action will help oneself (or some other person or persons) avoid or relieve some harm or gain some good. ("Goods" are abilities, freedom, opportunity, and pleasure.) Patients almost always make treatment decisions in order to avoid or ameliorate a harm rather than to gain a good, so goods do not frequently play a role in classifying patients' treatment decisions. Thus, if I believe that by enduring some pain (for example, having a bone marrow examination), I have an opportunity to avoid or postpone some other harm (death or serious disability from a possible leukemia), that belief is a reason for enduring the pain.

A reason is an *adequate reason* when at least some rational persons would agree that the harms avoided (or the goods gained) by suffering the harms of a contemplated act compensate for the harms caused by that act. Thus not all reasons are adequate reasons. Having a leg amputated to eliminate the mild pain caused by a plantar wart would count as a reason for the amputation, but it would not be an adequate reason, because no rational person would agree that the harms incurred by losing a leg are compensated for by the elimination of mild pain from the wart. However, having a leg amputated to try to stop the spread of an osteogenic sarcoma in the tibia would count as an adequate reason and would therefore be a rational treatment decision. The effect of having an adequate reason (for example, stopping the spread of cancer) is to turn an otherwise irrational action or decision (having a leg amputated) into a rational one.

In the case described, the patient's treatment refusal was irrational: He offered no reason for refusing the IV line, an action that had a significant probability of leading to his death. We would say he had no reason, certainly no adequate reason, using the definition of adequate reason given above, because he understood that ECT would relieve his suffering. We are not saying he had no *motive* for refusing; undoubtedly he did. But motives need not count as reasons, on the definition of "reason" given here.

We have now defined several terms in medical ethics and seen how they apply to this case.* The question can now be addressed: was it morally justified to start the IV against his wishes? We believe that it was, and this is reflected by the justification criteria enumerated above: 1) the harm the treatment might well avoid is very great (death); 2) the harms imposed by the IV treatment were, by comparison, very much less; 3) the patient's desire not to have the IV inserted was seriously irrational; 4) rational persons would, we believe, essentially always advocate allowing forced treatment in cases having the above three characteristics.

Acting Paternalistically Toward Persons with Psychiatric Disorders. The above analysis allows us to comment on an important question: What role does the presence of a psychiatric disorder have in justifying paternalistic actions directed toward the person with the disorder? On the face of it, no role at all. There is no mention in the above justification-of-paternalism criteria of the presence or absence of psychiatric disorders. It is true that persons with psychiatric disorders frequently have irrational desires not to be treated, and thus the third criterion is frequently satisfied, but satisfying that criterion alone does not justify forced paternalistic treatment.

What is critical is that the irrational desire not to be treated, which is often experienced by those with psychiatric disorders, is frequently transient; in particular it is true that if the person receives treatment, the irrational desire not to be treated often disappears fairly quickly. Thus, there is a good chance that the harms associated with the forced treatment (for example, the risks of the treatment, plus the mental pain associated with

---

*Several of these terms are discussed in more detail in the final chapter.

receiving a treatment one does not want) will not need to be inflicted for a very long time. Since the harms will therefore be less in extent, it is more likely that the paternalistic behavior will be morally justified than, say, similar paternalistic behavior directed toward a person whose irrational desires are not easily reversible. Thus, it is the reversibility of the irrational desires associated with psychiatric disorders that often plays an important role in justifying forced treatment of the mentally ill.

There is another important feature to point out about this case. We have advocated forced treatment of a patient whom we have described as competent but whose treatment refusal was seriously irrational. This is at variance with the belief held by some clinicians that only the presence of incompetence justifies forcing treatment on an unwilling patient. In most cases of forced treatment, this issue does not arise because most persons who make seriously irrational treatment refusals are, in fact, not fully competent. However, in occasional cases like this one, such patients are fully competent. These cases show that it is actually the irrationality of the refusal, and not the patient's competence (i.e., his ability to understand and appreciate relevant information) that accounts for our moral intuitions. When these cases arise, it is frequently necessary, as a legal safeguard, that the clinician go to court and have the patient declared "incompetent" before forced treatment may be carried out. In our experience, probate judges readily declare patients who make seriously irrational decisions incompetent even when the patients satisfy the definition of competence used here. This issue is discussed in more detail in the final chapter.

Discussion Questions

1. We believe that the ethically appropriate action in this case—to start the IV line—is reasonably uncontroversial: that essentially everyone would agree that that course of action was ethically justifiable. In the majority of instances of possible paternalistic actions, it does seem to be reasonably clear-cut that they either would or would not be ethically justifiable. How-

ever, there will inevitably be borderline, controversial cases as well. For example, suppose all the above facts about Mr. Brody are the same, but it is also true that he suffers from a lymphoma which is expected to kill him in two to three months. He refuses ECT and also the IV line. It is simply unclear in talking to him whether he is refusing treatment because of his depression or because he is terminally ill or because of some combination of the two. His family is unsure what should be done and asks Dr. Lynn what he thinks. Should the IV line be started? If this case seems less clear to you, can you think of a reasonable approach to take to borderline cases?

2. Residents sometimes do and sometimes do not identify themselves as trainees when they meet patients. If a resident introduces himself as "Dr. Young" and does not state that he is a resident, is that paternalistic behavior according to the above definition? Whether it is or is not, is it (ever) ethically justified for a resident not to reveal his or her trainee status?

References for Cases 6 and 7

Beauchamp, T. L., & Childress, J. F. (1989). *Principles of biomedical ethics* (3rd ed., pp. 209–227). New York: Oxford.

Culver, C. M., & Gert, B. (1982). *Philosophy in medicine* (pp. 126–163). New York: Oxford.

Sartorius, R. (Ed.) (1983). *Paternalism.* Minneapolis: University of Minnesota Press.

Thompson, D. F. (1987). *Political ethics and public office* (pp. 148–177). Cambridge, MA: Harvard University Press.

CASE 7. TREATING UNWILLING PATIENTS: SECOND CASE

Dr. Garcia of the psychiatric consultation service was asked to see a 68-year-old woman, Mrs. Elkin. It was her third admission to the hospital, and her attending internist was concerned that the patient might be schizophrenic. Mrs. Elkin had been followed in the medical clinic for over a year and had had two previous hospitalizations. She entered the hospital on this occasion because of an episode of hematemesis on the morning of admission. Her doctors during previous admissions had reported that she had hallucinations. She had been seen by a psychiatric consultant nine months previously who had recommended starting her on trifluoperazine, but the attending physician had felt it was not essential and the patient had never been given any psychotropic medication. The patient denied any previous psychiatric contacts and had had no psychiatric hospitalizations. The initial history was obtained from the patient and from her three sisters with whom she lived.

Dr. Garcia found Mrs. Elkins to be a pleasant elderly woman, lying in bed with an IV in her right arm and a cotton plug in each ear. When asked about the cotton plugs, she said, "Excuse yourself, don't press lip to tooth." Other comments were, "I'm listening to voices," "They are persons," and, "They are talking about lawyers." She said she sometimes had visions of "gentlemen" and "eyes." She indicated that sometimes the TV could control her thoughts. Except for this bizarre ideation, her speech was clear and coherent. She had taken the city bus to the hospital the morning of admission. She was oriented to person, place and time, and easily remembered three objects after five minutes. She was warm, related well, and was generally likeable and engaging.

Her sisters were of limited help with further history except to confirm that the patient had been hearing voices for about the past 10 years. Nonetheless, she was able to carry out most activities of daily living quite satisfactorily.

In sum, the patient appeared to be frankly psychotic, but had no evidence of any organic brain difficulty. Because of the late onset of her illness and the intactness of her ability to relate well with others, a firm diagnosis of schizophrenia could not be made. Dr. Garcia's tentative impression was Atypical Psychosis (in DSM-III-R: Psychotic Disorder Not Otherwise Specified).

She was shortly discharged because she was medically stable. She had refused transfer to the psychiatric service. At discharge, in addition to peptic ulcer medications, she was given haloperidol, 1 mg BID, and benztropine, 1 mg, to be taken BID if muscular stiffness developed. She gave what was judged by the psychiatrist to be a valid consent to taking these medications.

She was readmitted to the medical service one week later with the following history: Within two days of discharge she had felt dizzy and had some stiffness so she discontinued all medication. A few days later she developed nausea and vomiting, producing a significant degree of coffee ground-like material. The medical service believed that she was continuing to bleed from her ulcer, and that it was impossible to expect the patient to comply with taking medication. A surgical consultant recommended vagotomy and pyloroplasty but the patient refused, for unclear reasons. No one thought she was in any immediate danger from her bleeding ulcer, but in view of her noncompliance it was believed that surgery was the only viable long-range treatment option.

Dr. Garcia was again called and asked whether it would be appropriate to proceed with surgery against the patient's wishes. The surgical consultant placed great pressure on Dr. Garcia to declare the patient incompetent and to sanction his operating on her against her wishes and doing so as quickly as possible. Dr. Garcia specifically quizzed the surgeon about how much immediate danger existed for Mrs. Elkin; the surgeon admitted that waiting a few days would not result in a significantly increased risk.

When seen, Mrs. Elkin easily remembered Dr. Garcia. She was once again oriented to person, place and time. She continued to have auditory hallucinations. In addition she had developed delusions pertaining to her gastrointestinal problems. She confided to Dr. Garcia that she had been readmitted because of all the filth and blood she had vomited out of her system. She also thought that the blood she had vomited had been fed to her by someone. Despite repeated attempts, she either could not or would not say clearly why she would not consent to surgery. What should the consulting psychiatrist recommend?

Discussion

This patient's level of competence was not clear. She appeared to understand most of what she was told about the probable outcome of her condition with and without surgery, but her reluctance to discuss the subject made it difficult to measure her degree of understanding and appreciation. However, whether she was partially or fully competent, it was clear that she was consistently refusing the surgery.

Using the justification criteria given in Case 6, we do not believe it would be ethically justified to immediately override her refusal. It is true that her refusal of surgery was probably irrational. At least she was not able or willing to voice any reason, let alone an adequate one, for not choosing the one treatment that offered her significant hope of long-range relief from the harms associated with a bleeding ulcer. However, her medical condition without surgery was not sufficiently dangerous in the near future to balance the great amount of harm that would be perpetrated on her by forcing her to have an operation she did not desire. If there had been a high probability that she would die without immediate surgery, her refusal might have been seriously irrational; also, the harms of forced surgery would have been clearly outweighed by the prevention of her death. Under the latter circumstances, we believe that rational persons would agree that it would be universally allowable to carry out forced treatment in cases of this kind.

Because the patient was in little immediate danger, Dr. Garcia advised restarting haloperidol with the hope that Mrs. Elkin's mental status would improve to the point where it would be clearer whether she did understand and appreciate the information relevant to her situation. Also, she might be more disclosing about her reasons for refusing treatment. The patient agreed to take haloperidol once again. Several days later Mrs. Elkin said that she would be willing to have some more tests and, if Dr. Garcia could explain clearly to her that the tests indicated the need for surgery, she would agree.

Discussion Question

1. Suppose Mrs. Elkin had refused to take haloperidol again. What should Dr. Garcia advise? One thing he could advise would be not to force surgery on her against her wishes, but to

force haloperidol, perhaps via injection, in the hope it would have the above result. Would it be ethically justified to give her haloperidol against her wishes?

Reference (see also Case 6)

Applebaum, P. S. (1988). The right to refuse treatment with antipsychotic medications: Retrospect and prospect. *American Journal of Psychiatry, 145,* 413–419.

CASE 8. DETAINMENT OF A HOMELESS PERSON

A disheveled woman in her mid-40s was brought to the Emergency Department (ED) by the police at 3:00 a.m. on a Thursday morning. They requested that she be admitted to the psychiatry service. She was, so far as the police knew, homeless, and had been seen sleeping in a city park in recent months. She sometimes used the restroom at a nearby Burger King, but occasionally had been seen voiding amongst bushes in the park. The woman spent her days standing on street corners in the neighborhood and appeared to be hearing and responding to voices. She sometimes frightened pedestrians by yelling at them, but she did not appear truly menacing or dangerous. No one knew anything of her history. The police searched her satchel of belongings, which contained mostly clothes and ripped-out magazine articles. She had about $7.00 in cash and some candy. There was no evidence of legal or illegal drugs. The police had observed her culling food from neighborhood garbage cans.

The woman refused to give her name or to say more than a few words to Dr. Stinson, who examined her. She appeared reasonably well nourished and her vital signs were within normal limits. She would not give her name or say anything about her background. She seemed tense and frightened in the ED, and was obviously having almost continuous auditory hallucinations. She was very angry at one of the policemen, and periodically screamed and shook her fist at him. She refused to be admitted to the hospital or even to discuss taking medications. The police brought her in on this particular night because she had been screaming especially loudly for the past two nights, and several occupants of lower-floor apartments had called the police and complained. The policemen strongly urged Dr. Stinson to involuntarily hospitalize the woman.

Discussion

Cases like these are ethically difficult, and how best to manage the homeless mentally ill is an important social and psychiatric problem. It is an issue about which psychiatrists have much to say that is important, but it is not just a psychiatric issue. We will not try to offer a general solution to the problem here, but hope to show the nature of some important underlying conceptual and ethical issues.

Involuntary hospitalization is always an action that needs explicit ethical justification. It is important to be aware that this is so. Commitment statutes give the psychiatrist great power over the life of another person, power that can be exercised with limited review or due process for a period of time. In most states, a psychiatrist, on the force of her signature alone, can deprive another person of her freedom even if that person strongly desires not to be so deprived. It is not just deprivation of freedom but psychological pain that may be at stake. The patient may be manacled, whether dangerous-appearing or not, transported in a police car to a distant town, and held in a locked ward, which may be poorly staffed and filled with people who act in frightening ways. This deprivation of freedom is exempt from judicial review for two to three working days in most states; thus, a Friday detainment before a three-day weekend may not be reviewed, even if the court is punctual, until the next Wednesday or Thursday.

Thus detainment represents a significant impingement on the civil liberties of another person; the burden is on the psychiatrist to justify such an action ethically. However, it seems clear that in many cases detainment is ethically justified, and that in fact the psychiatrist would be acting unethically if she did not detain the patient.

Detainment is nearly always a paternalistic action. It clearly is that whenever we detain a patient to prevent her from possibly harming herself; even when the person is primarily acting menacingly to some other person, we usually believe with good reason that it is in the patient's best interest to be prevented from harming another, so detainment is almost always at least partially paternalistic.

The Justification of Detainment. When is paternalistic detainment ethically justified? The criteria for ethically justified paternalistic behavior given in Case 6 can be applied straightforwardly to detainment. Detainment inflicts certain harm on the patient: deprivation of freedom and, in almost all cases, mental suffering. However, it only probably prevents harm. It is rarely, if ever, certain that the harm one hopes to prevent would definitely occur if one did not detain. Thus, most observers agree that there must be a fairly high probability that detainment will prevent a very serious harm, such as death or permanent physical disability, before it can be ethically justified.

Many cases meet these criteria; for example, for a patient who is seriously suicidal and who is suffering from a transient, severe depression, the possibility of death seems relatively high, and, if the person is detained, the chance is very great that the person's mental illness can be successfully treated in a fairly short period of time. Thus, one would be inflicting harm relatively briefly in order probably to prevent irreversible harm of great magnitude. Most rational persons would agree that violating the moral rules against causing pain and depriving of freedom should be allowed in cases of this kind, and the paternalistic action therefore seems ethically justified.

However, the case of the homeless woman is more problematic. Although she clearly seems mentally ill, there is no evidence that she poses any immediate danger to herself or to other people. Yet psychiatrists can strongly desire to treat such persons. They appear to be ill; they often are clearly distraught and suffering from mental symptoms; there is a good chance that with treatment they would become less psychotic, feel happier, and be grateful that they had been treated. But many observers, especially persons who are not psychiatrists, do not feel forced treatment is justified. The harms from which the woman is suffering, as reversible as they may be, may not seem sufficiently severe to warrant the imposition of other serious harms on her, which she explicitly rejects. While the woman's desire not to be treated is arguably irrational, it may not be sufficiently irrational to justify overruling her wishes.

The Prediction of Dangerousness. An important issue raised by detainment is the extent to which psychiatrists are validly able to predict that particular individuals will on particular occasions act in a dangerous way. Few psychiatrists, even those whose threshold for detainment is high and who detain only the most intensely ill and homicidal and/or suicidal patients, believe that everyone they detain would, if not detained, carry out those actions which detainment is intended to prevent.

There are few data available about what fraction of those detained are indeed prevented from harming themselves or others. Such data are, for obvious reasons, difficult to obtain, but the underlying issue is important to consider. Suppose, for example, that three out of four depressed, suicidal patients would kill themselves without detainment. Most people would probably feel detainment was morally justified, even though one of the four patients was unnecessarily detained. However, suppose only 1 in 100 of those detained would commit suicide. Most would probably feel it unjustified to deprive 99 people of their freedom unnecessarily in order to save one life. The actual fraction is unknown, though some estimates have been about one in five or one in six. If true, four or five people are being unnecessarily deprived of their freedom in order to save one person.

One important point to note is that the one to five or one to six ratio may be the best that psychiatrists can do, at least at present. This is because it is difficult to predict rare events without making many "false positive" predictions, that is, predicting that something will happen when in fact it will not. False positives are frequent even when the tests available are very accurate, as will be noted in a later case which discusses HIV testing. When the tests are less accurate, as are the signs and symptoms that can be noted in the ED with a suicidal patient, the false positive problem is great.

Discussion Questions

1. Suppose actuarial tables were available which correlated with some precision the signs and symptoms a patient displayed in the ED with his probability of killing himself if not detained, and that one could assign any particular patient to a cohort. Further, suppose one patient had a 1 in 3 chance of killing himself, but another patient had only a 1 in 12 chance. If you were not a psychiatrist, but a member of a group of rational persons deciding what ratio you wanted the psychiatrists in your midst to use, what ratio would you choose? What logical justification can be offered for choosing any particular ratio over the next significantly higher or lower ones?

2. Some observers feel that in recent decades the legislative pendulum has swung too far and that the criteria for detainment in most states are too narrow. Persons of this opinion may argue, for example, that requiring that a mentally ill patient be "immediately physically dangerous to himself or others" is too restrictive and that all that should be required is that the patient suffer from "serious psychological dysfunction." Other observers disagree and favor the narrower criteria. What empirical data, if any, could be collected which might help resolve this dispute, and how would you go about obtaining them?

References

Chodoff, P. (1976). The case for involuntary hospitalization of the mentally ill. *American Journal of Psychiatry, 133,* 496–501.

Culver, C. M., & Gert, B. (1982). *Philosophy in medicine* (pp. 146–178). New York: Oxford.

Glasser, I. (1978). Power versus liberty in the welfare state. In W. Gaylin, I. Glasser, S. Marcus, & D. Rothman (Eds.), *Doing good: The limits of benevolence* (pp. 97–168). New York: Pantheon.

Livermore, J. M., Malmquist, C. P., & Meehl, P. E. (1968). On the justification for civil commitment. *University of Pennsylvania Law Review, 117,* 75–96.

Roth, L. (1979). A commitment law for patients, doctors, and lawyers. *American Journal of Psychiatry, 136,* 1121–1127.

CASE 9. THE SUICIDE OF A PATIENT AFTER A JUDGMENT NOT TO DETAIN

Mr. Shea, a 54-year-old, divorced male lawyer, with a long history of bipolar affective disorder, was brought to the Emergency Department (ED) on a Saturday afternoon by his 24-year-old son. Mr. Shea was a resident of a neighboring state and was visiting his son for the weekend. His son had initiated the visit to the ED out of concern that his father seemed more depressed than he had for some time. Dr. Snyder, the on-call psychiatry resident, talked with Mr. Shea and his son at some length. She determined that Mr. Shea had indeed been depressed for the past several weeks and had resumed seeing his at-home psychiatrist, Dr. Higgins, who had cared for him for many years. Dr. Higgins had started him on some antidepressant medication, which Mr. Shea said was already making him feel better. Nonetheless, Mr. Shea's son was worried and urged Dr. Snyder to admit his father to the hospital.

On examination by Dr. Snyder, Mr. Shea appeared to be moderately depressed. He did not appear agitated, and he denied suicidal ideation or intent. He firmly refused to enter the hospital. He acknowledged that he was depressed, but said he was already feeling better since seeing Dr. Higgins and starting to take medication. He said, "I've been this route many times before." He minimized his son's concern, saying his son had rarely been around him when he had the "blues."

Dr. Snyder would have admitted Mr. Shea to the local psychiatry unit if the patient were willing, but he clearly was not. The only way to hospitalize him would be to detain him and have the police escort him to the state hospital 30 miles away. She did not feel that detainment was clinically indicated. Mr. Shea seemed to be functioning reasonably well at home and at work, and neither the patient nor his son reported any signs or symptoms that suggested a particular danger of suicidality. Thus, not only was detainment not clinically indicated, but Mr. Shea did not fulfill the legal criteria for detainment in the state. These required the presence of a major mental disorder, which Mr. Shea did have, and the presence of a clear risk of danger to self or others, of which there was no compelling evidence.

With Mr. Shea's permission, Dr. Snyder called Dr. Higgins and luckily was able to reach him at home. After hearing Dr. Snyder's observations, Dr. Higgins agreed that the situation did not appear to warrant detainment. Dr. Higgins stated that he had seen Mr. Shea this depressed or even somewhat worse on several occasions, that he had never appeared or acted suicidal, and that he usually responded well to the medication he was now taking.

After discussing the situation over the phone with her back-up attending psychiatrist, who concurred with her judgment, Dr. Snyder allowed the patient to leave. She told the patient and his son to call her anytime over the next two days or nights if the situation changed. She obtained the son's telephone number and said that she would call on Sunday to see how Mr. Shea was feeling. She thoroughly documented the clinical interaction and the reasons for her actions in a note in Mr. Shea's chart. Mr. Shea and his son returned to the son's house. Two hours later Mr. Shea died of a self-inflicted gunshot wound.

Discussion

The outcome of this case was tragic, but it does not follow that Dr. Snyder acted clinically incorrectly or without ethical justification. While any moderately depressed patient is probably at greater risk of suicide than a nondepressed randomly selected person, the risk does not seem sufficiently high in cases like Mr. Shea's to warrant forced hospitalization. Suppose that persons presenting like Mr. Shea later kill themselves in 1 out of 100 cases. We believe that most rational persons would agree that 1 out of 100 is not a sufficiently high ratio to justify the serious and certain harms which accompany the paternalistic act of detainment.

No matter where one draws the general line above which one will not commit, there will inevitably be occasional cases that fall above this line who go on and harm themselves. It is not just likely, it is certain this will occur: 1 out of 100 is 1 out of 100, it is not 0 out of 100. If a psychiatrist in full-time outpatient practice never in his career has a patient who kills himself, he may be detaining too many patients. The situation is analogous to general surgeons operating for presumptive appendicitis: The surgeon who never finds a normal appendix at laporotomy is probably not operating often enough. The surgeon, like the psychiatrist, is balancing harms caused (by general anesthesia, etc.) with harms possibly prevented (rupture, peritonitis, possible death). A general line is drawn above and below which one will or will not operate with the realization that neither decision will always prove to be correct.

Whether an action is ethically justified or not depends on the facts that one knows or should know at the time of the action, not on what the later outcome of the situation is. It is natural in cases like Mr. Shea's to wish one had done otherwise. It would not be surprising if Dr. Snyder engaged in considerable self-recrimination, perhaps blaming herself for not listening more to the patient's son. Her back-up attending psychiatrist might blame himself for not having come in to the ED to examine the patient personally, though this was not required in this program. No matter what Dr. Snyder had read about indications for detainment, no matter how supportive her colleagues might be, her self-confidence might well be shaken. But although she feels badly she should be reassured by her supervisors and colleagues that she has made a reasonable and quite defensible professional judgment.

Discussion Questions

1. Do you agree that if only 1 in 100 persons detained would later commit serious self-harm, that detainment would be ethically unjustified? Suppose someone disagreed, saying she felt that saving even one life justified detaining 99 persons who would not have harmed themselves if not detained. What arguments could be given against her position? How might she reply?

2. Suppose that, by bizarre coincidence, Dr. Snyder is on-call two months later when a depressed patient comes to the ED, accompanied by his family, in circumstances eerily similar to Mr. Shea's. What should Dr. Snyder do differently?

4

RELATIONSHIPS WITH COLLEAGUES

CASE 10. THE RESIDENT'S ROLE IN DECISION-MAKING

For the past six months, a 25-year-old man, Mr. Stein, had been engaged in psychodynamic, insight-oriented psychotherapy with a third-year resident, Dr. Fry, for an obsessive-compulsive disorder (OCD). The psychotherapy, which was supervised by a senior psychiatrist, Dr. Baird, had led to the patient's becoming less inhibited at work and had also been an excellent learning experience for the resident. However, there had been no change in Mr. Stein's presenting complaints of obsessive rumination, ritualistic cleaning behaviors, and compulsive checking of details.

During a psychopharmacology seminar, Dr. Fry learned that a particular drug, clomipramine, had been found to be of definite benefit to many patients suffering from OCD. Dr. Fry described Mr. Stein's symptoms to the leader of the seminar, who suggested that Dr. Fry give Mr. Stein a trial of clomipramine.

Dr. Fry felt an immediate sense of conflict at this suggestion. It had become obvious during supervision that Dr. Baird adopted a purely psychological view of the etiology and treatment of OCD. Dr. Fry was reluctant to do anything that might cause his influential supervisor to question his clinical judgment. Beyond this concrete concern, he was anxious to be liked and respected by a senior clinician whose own excellence was acknowledged by everyone in the department. Suggesting a therapeutic direction that Dr. Baird did not consider appropriate might cause his supervisor to question his competence as a psychotherapist.

Thus, Dr. Fry foresaw serious potential problems in even discussing OCD medication with his supervisor. He considered several options. One was to proceed with psychotherapy and ignore the possibility of using medication. After all, Mr. Stein was involved in therapy and had made some small gains. But Dr. Fry rejected this option: It would leave Mr. Stein himself unaware of the possibility of trying medication, a choice he might well favor since, in truth, his presenting complaints were essentially unchanged. A second option would be to recommend a medication trial to Mr. Stein, but continue at the same time with psychotherapy, and not tell Dr. Baird about the medication. But this seemed a poor choice also: It would have introduced a major deceptive element into the supervisory relationship. Finally Dr. Fry decided the best course was the honest course: Discuss with Dr. Baird the possibility of treating Mr. Stein with a combined psychotherapy-medication approach.

Dr. Fry felt caught between the practical need to be viewed in a positive light by a supervisor who could strongly influence his career, and the ethical requirement to practice psychiatry competently. In psychiatry, competent (and thus ethical) practice involves understanding different and occasionally even contradictory conceptualizations of the same disorder. Even when it is not possible to integrate psychological and biological treatment approaches fully at a conceptual level, it may be necessary to consider using both with particular patients.

Therefore, Dr. Fry decided to address the question of supplemental medication directly with Dr. Baird. Dr. Baird responded by complimenting Dr. Fry on his thoroughness, but he was convinced that even raising the possibility of medication would be experienced by the patient as a message that he had failed in therapy. Dr. Baird believed that no matter how objectively the question of medication were raised, Mr. Stein would interpret it as a sign of the therapist's lack of confidence in the patient's ability to solve his own problems, much as his mother used to control various aspects of his life that she believed he could not control for himself. Dr. Fry once again faced a dilemma about how he should proceed.

One alternative was simply to follow Dr. Baird's advice. Dr. Baird was knowledgeable about Mr. Stein's psychopathology. Since for this particular patient he bore both clinical and supervisory responsibility, he was responsible for Mr. Stein's treatment. He might have positive feelings toward a resident who responded well to his suggestions. But Dr. Fry finally decided he could not follow this course: It left Mr. Stein out of the decision-making process.

It is not necessary or even possible that a psychiatrist be able to administer all types of treatment, but a competent psychiatrist should know about the important ones and be able to describe their respective merits and drawbacks to his patients. The choice of treatments is ultimately the patient's, though the psychiatrist is free to give the patient his advice. The patient's choice cannot be made knowledgeably and therefore validly, as discussed earlier, unless the patient is aware of the range of treatments available. It is not correct to assume that because a patient has entered a particular type of treatment, the patient must desire that treatment only; the patient may be simply uninformed about the other available options.

Dr. Fry decided on the following course of action, to which Dr. Baird, after a long discussion, agreed. He informed the patient about the possibility of taking clomipramine, and also about taking other medications that have been used to treat OCD. The patient, as expected, became obsessively preoccupied about making a choice, but this proved to be a useful reaction to examine in psychotherapy. It became apparent that the resident's and the supervisor's reluctance to inform the patient about drug treatment of OCD reflected in part an identification with the patient's reluctance to take responsibility for himself. The patient initially insisted that the physician decide for him; working through this wish with the patient proved more therapeutic than acting out the patient's lack of confidence in his ability to decide for himself.

The patient did decide on a trial of clomipramine, but the medication was not helpful. However, the experience of making a definite decision made him feel motivated to deal more forcefully with other difficult decisions. He eventually took another medication, fluoxetine, which did relieve some of his obsessive and compulsive symptoms. Psychotherapy was facilitated because patient and therapist had to be less preoccupied with these disabling and time-consuming symptoms. Both Dr. Fry and Dr. Baird felt they had learned something valuable in the process of working through this case.

Discussion

This case had a happy ending; not all similar cases do. Residents are sometimes caught in the middle between the competing treatment orientations of their supervisors. It is inevitable and not entirely disadvantageous that senior psychiatrists become personally invested in their own areas of greatest knowledge and competence. Not everyone can do everything well, and the presence of skilled and dedicated role models, even ones with narrow orientations, can be a plus for a training program. What is important is that the department have an explicit norm that encourages questioning and challenging. The university should be one place where open discussion and disagreement is expected, even welcomed. And where professionals disagree about the most appropriate therapy in a given setting, it should almost always be the patient who elects which course to take.

Discussion Question

1. Suppose Dr. Baird had continued to insist that Mr. Stein not be told about the possibility of drug therapy. Does Dr. Fry have an ethical duty to do anything further? What steps might he take? At what point, if any, should he involve his Training Director in the situation?

CASE 11. IMPAIRMENT IN A COLLEAGUE

Dr. Janeway, a third-year resident, considered herself lucky to have Dr. Kroll as a supervisor. Dr. Kroll was one of the most respected senior faculty members in the Department of Psychiatry. Not only was he capable of perceiving the most subtle psychopathological nuances in Dr. Janeway's patients, he knew a great deal about current drug therapies.

Dr. Janeway had been particularly impressed with Dr. Kroll's insight and knowledge during their first supervisory session. She was surprised during the next session that he had forgotten many important details of the case they had been discussing. She decided that he must simply be having a bad day, but over the next few sessions his performance as a supervisor was even more erratic. At one point, she was certain that there was a strong smell of alcohol on his breath.

Dr. Janeway felt conflicted. Although Dr. Kroll's supervision was proving unpredictable, it was obvious that he had a great deal to teach. Even so, his performance as a supervisor appeared to have deteriorated from a level that previously must have been far higher. Dr. Janeway wondered whether Dr. Kroll's impairment had been evident but had been minimized by other supervisees and peers. Was his reputation based more on past achievements than present abilities? More importantly, if Dr. Kroll was having so much trouble keeping track of well-organized material presented during supervision, how was this busy practitioner functioning as a clinician? Did she have a responsibility to address these questions personally?

Discussion

Dealing with impaired or possibly impaired colleagues raises many important ethical, legal and practical issues. It is true, except in the rarest of cases, that physicians should put patients' interests above all other matters, certainly above the comfort of physicians. Because physicians have this responsibility toward all patients, the benefit of protecting any future patients from substandard care outweighs the harm caused to a colleague's reputation if impairment is unavoidably revealed. Physicians who are impaired should be treated aggressively, and, in those rare instances where their underlying disorder is not treatable, they should be prevented from continuing to practice medicine.

In fact, balancing harms and benefits and deciding how to proceed is often easier when dealing with impaired physicians than when facing other ethical dilemmas. This is because it is frequently not harmful on balance, even to the physician himself, to uncover and confront the impairment. Left to their own devices, many impaired physicians will not seek help early in the course of their illnesses. Not confronting the problem may enhance the physician's denial, and the illness may become more and more dangerous to the physician and his patients. There is excellent evidence that many forms of impairment, especially those caused by acute psychiatric illness and by substance abuse, can be very effectively treated.

Unfortunately, many physicians are reluctant to confront their impaired colleagues. This seems especially true in situations like Dr. Janeway's, where the impaired colleague has the kind of reputation, seniority or authority that makes a junior colleague doubt whether anything could actually be wrong. Also, many physicians are uncomfortable at the thought of a confrontation, or believe that the possibility that another doctor has a problem is none of their business.

Section 2 of the American Medical Association's *Principles of Medical Ethics* makes the obligation to take action explicit: "A physician shall deal honestly with patients and colleagues, and strive to expose those physicians deficient in character or competence, or who engage in fraud or deception." (See Appendix.) To ensure that physicians carry out that ethical obligation, some states have even enacted laws stipulating that the license of a physician with knowledge of a colleague's impairment may be in jeopardy if the physician does not report that colleague to a licensing body.

Many states have an independent body, such as an impaired physician committee of the state medical society, that has the capacity to investigate allegations of impairment. If the allegation proves founded, a contract is sometimes established in which the physician agrees to evaluation and treatment, to the monitoring of his treatment and, where appropriate, to the monitoring of his clinical practice. The physician's medical license can be suspended if treatment is terminated prematurely or if there is a relapse into impaired performance. If treatment is terminated prematurely, in violation of a contract with the medical society's impaired physician committee, the physician must be reported to the state licensing board. Otherwise, treatment is kept confidential from the licensing board. There is good evidence that "contingency contracting" of this kind can be effective. Requiring an impaired colleague to seek treatment can therefore be beneficial both to the physician and to the physician's present and future patients.

We believe that the benefit of identifying fellow physicians who are impaired, regardless of their rank or stature, far outweighs the harm of exposing them and ourselves to embarrassment and anxiety. It can be a gratifying if somewhat tense experience to discuss one's observations with an impaired colleague, and allow that individual to seek appropriate treatment and take any necessary steps to protect any patients or trainees who might be injured by his impairment. If the impaired physician is unable or unwilling to acknowledge the problem or have it treated, a confidential report should be made to the appropriate official board and/or administrative authority. Any psychiatrist who is unsure whether his observations of a colleague actually indicate impairment, or is not sure how to proceed, should not hesitate to seek consultation from a colleague to help resolve the dilemma. Residents should always discuss the situation with their Training Director or, if for some reason that is not appropriate, with the departmental chairperson.

Discussion Question

1. Do you believe that Dr. Janeway has enough evidence at this point to take any action? If so, how specifically should she proceed?

Reference

Scheiber, S. C., & Doyle, B. B. (1983). *The impaired physician.* New York: Plenum.

CASE 12. SIGNING BLANK PRESCRIPTION FORMS

Dr. Reddy works one day a week at a Community Mental Health Center. The clinic could use two or three times more psychiatrists' hours, but they are glad to have Dr. Reddy even one day a week. It has proved difficult to recruit psychiatrists because of the clinic's rural location and low salary schedule. The clinic is staffed primarily by nonmedical mental health clinicians who have worked together for many years. They know their patients well and often in the past have had to function without any psychiatrist. When necessary, a local internist has, quite reluctantly, prescribed psychotropic medications.

Dr. Reddy provides a variety of services at the clinic. When he first arrives a team meeting is held during which new patients are discussed and treatment plans are proposed. Dr. Reddy signs the plans as per clinic requirements. Although he does not interview these patients himself, he has confidence in the staff's ability to obtain information and develop working diagnoses and treatment plans. Dr. Reddy then sees several patients who are referred for evaluation for medication. He also signs prescriptions for refills for patients he has evaluated and begun on medications in the past, but he does not generally see them in person. If there is a likelihood that these latter patients may need a future change in their dose, he leaves the dosage blank to be filled in by the clinician who knows the patient best. He assumes that if the clinician has any questions, he will be consulted.

Finally, he signs his name on the third party billing forms prepared by social work clinicians who cannot bill directly. If he has any serious concerns about the treatment being provided by a social worker, these are discussed before the forms are signed. Otherwise, the forms are simply submitted with his signature.

Dr. Reddy is a dedicated and competent psychiatrist, but the ethical dimensions of his actions deserve scrutiny. Should he sign treatment plans for patients he has not seen? Should he prescribe medication for patients he evaluated initially but has not seen for several months? Should he give nonmedical clinicians the discretion to adjust the dosages of medications? Dr. Reddy is employed for only eight hours each week and himself would not be able to spend more time there. If he did not work at the clinic, it is unlikely they would be able to find another psychiatrist. Few psychiatrists are available in the area, and most of them would not work for the salary that is provided. Do the benefits of meeting the needs of the clinic as best he can with the time available ethically justify the practices in which Dr. Reddy engages?

Discussion

The American Psychiatric Association (1989) has suggested a set of guidelines for "signing off" in cases like the one described. These guidelines were approved by the APA's Board of Trustees in June 1989.

While the physician's signature indicates that he or she is legally and ethically responsible for the action or consequences of the document signed, the guidelines suggest that there can be degrees of this responsibility. The first three of these APA guidelines follow:

> 1. The signature of a psychiatrist on a diagnostic formulation or treatment plan signifies that the psychiatrist has reviewed, agreed with the diagnosis, and approved of the plan. This does not necessarily mean that he or she has seen the patient or carried out the evaluation. It may imply only that he or she is head or a member of a multidisciplinary team or supervisor of other professionals or trainees. The psychiatrist should clarify his or her role in the process of the formulation by writing immediately before his or her signature "Reviewed by [name]" or "Under the supervision of [name]" or "Team Leader Approval" or other clarification.

2. The initiation of pharmacologic treatment by a psychiatrist will require the direct evaluation of the patient. This should include a comprehensive review of relevant history—medical, psychiatric, and previous response to medication. There may be circumstances where a direct evaluation is not possible at the time of prescription or order. In this case, evaluation should be completed in a timely fashion. Maintenance of medication regimes also requires periodic direct reevaluation of the patient.

3. The signature of a psychiatrist on an insurance or other third-party form for billing purposes signifies that the patient has received the treatment for which the third party is being billed. Wording on the form must be carefully scrutinized to assure that the information is accurate. The psychiatrist is obligated to correct any errors or misconceptions since he or she will be held responsible. The psychiatrist should make clear on the form precisely the services that he or she is claiming and whether and to what extent he or she has directly treated or evaluated the patient. This obligation may be met by writing in before the signature a phrase such as "Under the supervision of [name]" or "Reviewed by [name]" or "Approved by [name]." The psychiatrist may also review the patient's record or require additional information to insure the accuracy of the diagnosis and the services being billed for have been documented. (p. 1390)

Are Dr. Reddy's actions in accordance with these guidelines? How clear are the guidelines about prescribing practices?

We believe there is a definite clinical risk and therefore an ethical concern if Dr. Reddy leaves signed prescription forms that are blank in any respect. He cannot be certain who will use them and under what circumstances. Additionally, even dedicated nonmedical clinicians are rarely if ever sufficiently knowledgeable to investigate patients' use of other medications or the development of unusual symptoms or side effects.

Dr. Reddy might consider using nonpsychiatrist physicians in the community as resources. They could monitor many patients' courses on medication, using him as a consultant, and he could personally evaluate nonresponding patients and those with more complex problems. The clinic might well be willing to pay for the few additional hours of medical time this would require, and such a plan would utilize Dr. Reddy's skills and availability better than the present one.

Dr. Reddy may feel too inexperienced administratively to challenge the clinic's practices. He should meet with the director and clarify his ethical and legal responsibilities and set appropriate limits, remembering that his first responsibility is to the welfare of his patients. The existence of the above APA guidelines may be helpful to him, since he could argue that it would be unethical and imprudent of him to practice in a way counter to APA recommendations. While one could argue that even an implied threat to resign from the clinic staff might create some possibility of leaving this group of patients without any psychiatric care, the fear of losing him could be a catalyst for change in a more clinically appropriate direction.

Discussion Questions

1. Do you think it is ever possible for a psychiatrist to assume meaningful responsibility for a patient whom he or she has not personally examined? Is it possible to approve of a treatment plan in an ethically justified way without a personal examination? If you think it sometimes is possible and sometimes is not, how would you describe the difference?

2. Can you think of one or more "signing off" situations the APA's first guideline does not cover with sufficient precision to enable one to know just what the guideline would recommend? If so, how could the guideline be written to give clearer and more precise ethical guidance?

References

American Psychiatric Association. (1980). Guidelines for psychiatrists in consultative, supervisory, or collaborative relationships with nonmedical therapists. *American Journal of Psychiatry, 137,* 1489–1491.

American Psychiatric Association. (1989). Guidelines regarding psychiatrists' signatures. *American Journal of Psychiatry, 146,* 1390.

5

SEXUAL ATTRACTION TOWARD PATIENTS

CASE 13. SEXUAL ATTRACTION TOWARD ONE'S OWN PATIENT

Dr. Hospers was a 30-year-old unmarried male resident. He realized he was becoming attracted to one of his women patients. She was a single, rather shy high-school teacher in her late 20s who suffered from a situational depression. He had seen her once weekly for about three months and therapy seemed to be progressing nicely. He realized he was thinking of her more and more often during his spare time, and although the subject hasn't yet come up in therapy, he was sure that she was attracted to him as well.

He wondered if it would be wrong to suggest to her that the two of them see each other socially on occasion. Both of them were single, and neither were involved with anyone else at the time. She seemed mature and not at all fragile—not like the women patients with whom he was aware some male doctors had become involved.

He thought, "I probably shouldn't do it. On the other hand, we would make a terrific couple. If we had met in a social setting, I'm sure we would have had a great relationship from the start. Why should the two of us be penalized because we had the ironic bad luck to meet under these circumstances? I'm a doctor, but more basically I'm a man; she's a patient, but more basically she's a woman. She doesn't really have any serious psychiatric illness at all, and if we did hit it off she could probably just drop out of therapy or else see someone else after a while if she needed to."

Discussion

Having sexual feelings toward patients is common. All therapists on occasion have sexual feelings, fantasies and/or dreams about their patients. The therapeutic encounter is marked by repetitive close contact, often great psychological intimacy, and an encouragement for the patient to be spontaneous and unguarded about what she or he is feeling and thinking. Both parties may feel on occasion the full gamut of emotions which two persons may have toward one another.

But while it is common for a therapist to have sexual feelings toward a patient, it almost always is harmful for both parties if these feelings are openly expressed. Even if it seems, ahead of time, that this will not be true, even if the therapist and the patient reassure each other that they will be able to manage a romantic or sexual relationship, it almost never turns out other than badly. The evidence for this is more anecdotal than empirical, but it is strong. Perhaps the two parties would have had a good relationship had they met socially, but they have not met socially. No matter how "mature" the patient is, the feelings she has for the therapist are inevitably colored by transferential elements that make the relationship unlike a social relationship. Though a romantic relationship between them might be initially pleasurable, the aftermath for the patient is almost always filled with pain, anger toward the therapist, and loathing toward herself.

It is so likely that great pain will result for both parties that it is unethical and irrational for the therapist to allow the relationship to become romantic or sexual. It is unethical because it is so likely to hurt the patient; less important, but still important, it is irrational because it is also likely to hurt the therapist.

It is not a mitigating factor if the initiative to form a personal relationship comes from the patient. Even if the patient is seductive and romantically aggressive, it is the psychiatrist's responsibility to maintain a professional distance in the relationship; almost always, in fact, the patient's seductiveness should be confronted in therapy as a manifestation of the transference.

We have said that romantic relationships "almost always" hurt the patient, but that "without question" (i.e., always) it would be unethical for the therapist to proceed. The slight distinction is intended. There may be rare occasions when neither the therapist nor the patient would be severely harmed by having a romantic relationship. But the probability of harm is so great that it is unethical to take the chance. There is general agreement that whether an action is ethical is determined not by what consequences do occur, but by what the probable consequences are at the time of the action. Loading half the cartridges into a gun, randomly twirling the chamber, and shooting at someone is a seriously unethical action even if by good fortune the other person is not harmed.

The case describes a male therapist and a female patient. That is the most frequent kind of case which occurs, both according to questionnaire surveys of therapists, and according to the kinds of ethics complaints lodged with District Branch Ethics Committees of the American Psychiatric Association. However, women therapists become involved with male patients as well, and homosexual liaisons also occur.

The resident in this case realized that it was generally wrong to become romantically involved with patients, but believed that in this particular instance, there were special mitigating factors. That is a belief therapists not infrequently possess before they become sexually involved with patients. Sexual feelings and needs are enormously powerful, and self-deception may be as frequent in this area as it is in the addictions. Feeling that anything at all about one's relationship with a particular patient is "special" should be a warning flag.

The best antidote to an emerging sexual interest in a patient is a frank and open discussion with one's Training Director, a supervisor, some other senior psychiatrist, or a personal therapist. It is surprising how effective even one session can be in decreasing the likelihood of becoming sexually involved. If discussion or supervision is not effective in controlling one's fear of sexual involvement with a patient, personal therapy may be necessary. At any rate, this is an issue that should be discussed with at least one supervisor as it is worked through.

There is nearly unanimous agreement among psychiatrists that a romantic or sexual relationship with a patient currently in therapy is almost always harmful and is always unethical. What about relationships with former patients? There is disagreement within the profession on this point and there are strong feelings on each side. Some feel that "once a patient, always a patient," that the deep, transferential elements of the relationship persist forever, and that romantic relationships should forever be forbidden. Others, though they agree that in most cases an ex-patient is as vulnerable and as likely to be harmed as a current patient, feel that there are cases in which the probability of harm is not as high, and believe that cases of ex-patients need to be considered individually. No one considers a patient within a few months after termination to be an ex-patient; the disagreement, rather, is whether there are rare cases in which a personal relationship commences some years after therapy has ended that might not necessarily represent unethical behavior on the part of the psychiatrist.

All psychiatrists should be aware of the American Psychiatric Association's guidelines on these matters. Section 2, Annotation 1, of *The Principles of Medical Ethics with Annotations Especially Applicable to Psychiatry* (APA, 1986; last sentence of following annotation approved by APA Trustees in December, 1988) reads as follows:

> The requirement that the physician conduct himself with propriety in his/her profession and in all the actions of his/her life is especially important in the case of the psychiatrist because the patient tends to model his/her behavior after that of his/her therapist by identification. Further, the necessary intensity of the therapeutic relationship may tend to activate sexual and other needs and fantasies on the part of both patient and therapist, while weakening the objectivity necessary for control. Sexual activity with a patient is unethical. Sexual involvement with one's former patients generally exploits emotions deriving from treatment and therefore almost always is unethical. (p. 4)

Discussion Questions

1. If it is true that on rare occasions romantic relationships with ex-patients are not unethical, what criteria should be used to determine which ones? If a psychiatrist did want to see an ex-patient socially and did not want to hurt her, or at least subject her to more risks than dating relationships usually have, are there any safeguards that could be taken ahead of time? Or do you believe, contra the APA's guidelines, that it is best simply to have a categorical rule always making it unethical to have a relationship with an ex-patient, no matter what the circumstances, and that the same sanctions should be levied against the psychiatrist as would be the case if the relationship involved a patient currently in treatment?

2. Some psychiatrists have married persons who have been their patients. Sometimes the romantic relationship began when the person was a current patient. What action, if any, should the profession take in these cases? If you believe no action should be taken, how do you explain the seeming paradox?

3. The APA (1986) has recently added the following to Section 4 of the *Annotation* booklet:

> Sexual involvement between a faculty member or supervisor and a trainee or student, in those situations in which an abuse of power can occur, often takes advantage of inequalities in the working relationship and may be unethical because: (a) any treatment of a patient being supervised may be deleteriously affected; (b) it may damage the trust relationship between teacher and student; and (c) teachers are important professional role models for their trainees and affect their trainees' future professional behavior. (p. 7)

Under what circumstances, if any, do you believe it is ethically justified for a supervisor and a supervisee to engage in a sexual relationship?

References

American Psychiatric Association. (1986). *The principles of medical ethics with annotations especially applicable to psychiatry.* Washington, DC: APA.

Gabbard, G. O. (Ed.) (1989). *Sexual exploitation in professional relationships.* Washington, DC: American Psychiatric Press.

Gartrell, N., Herman, J., Olarte, S., Localio, R., & Feldstein, M. (1988). Psychiatric residents' sexual contact with educators and patients: Results of a national survey. *American Journal of Psychiatry, 145,* 690–694.

Pope, K. S., Keith-Spiegel, P., & Tabachnick, B. G. (1986). Sexual attraction to clients. The human therapist and the (sometimes) inhuman training system. *American Psychologist, 41,* 147–158.

CASE 14. A PATIENT'S SEXUAL ACTIVITY WITH A FORMER THERAPIST

Dr. Youngfield was consulted by Mrs. Lawrence, a 28-year-old married woman who complained of constant anxiety, frequent headaches, and a sense of lack of fulfillment. She was a shy and intense woman who blushed frequently and only at the third interview revealed that she and her husband were having sexual difficulties. She had always been inhibited about sexual involvement. She rarely had an orgasm and admitted that she often used her psychological symptoms to avoid sexual activity with her husband. It was not until several sessions later that she revealed that she had had sexual intercourse with her previous psychiatrist, Dr. Oldham. He had told her that this would be beneficial for her sexual difficulties.

The patient had "fallen in love" with Dr. Oldham several weeks after they began having sex during her therapy hours. It soon became clear that while Dr. Oldham told her he cared very much for her, he had no intention of becoming permanently involved with her and certainly would not leave his family. She became enraged, then very depressed, and abruptly discontinued therapy. She had been without psychiatric help for over a year before seeing Dr. Youngfield and had told no one what had happened. She felt disgraced and ashamed.

Dr. Youngfield knew that having sexual relations with patients was categorically labeled as unethical by the American

Psychiatric Association (and by all other mental health professional associations). He knew also that he had a general duty to report unethical behavior on the part of a colleague to his local District Branch Ethics Committee of the APA. But he also knew that what Mrs. Lawrence had told him was confidential unless she gave him permission to tell others.

Dr. Youngfield told Mrs. Lawrence that Dr. Oldham's behavior was in violation of the American Psychiatric Association's Code of Ethics. He discussed with her what she wanted to do and described some available options. He told Mrs. Lawrence that if she wished to report Dr. Oldham to the local District Branch, he would be glad to assist her in finding out whom to call to initiate a complaint. However, she insisted that she was too ashamed of what happened to let anyone else know what had happened. Even the thought of lodging a complaint upset her a great deal.

Dr. Youngfield did not want to cause his patient further distress, but it was important to try to prevent future episodes of this kind by Dr. Oldham. Dr. Youngfield also thought it might in the long run help Mrs. Lawrence if she could bring herself to lodge a complaint. However, he was afraid that continuing to focus on this issue in their sessions, in the face of her continued refusal to report Dr. Oldham, might interfere with her therapy.

Dr. Youngfield thought of another possible course of action. He knew that there were, in the area, several senior psychiatrists who were willing to consult in these situations. He asked Mrs. Lawrence if she would be willing to talk about the options available to her with another psychiatrist before she made a final decision about reporting. He assured her that this second psychiatrist would be someone with experience in these matters, that he could explain in detail the various actions she could take, that in no way would he pressure her to take any particular course of action, and that she would be entirely free after the talk to continue to do nothing at all. She agreed to have such a talk.

She saw Dr. Casey. He explained that she had many options. They lived in a state that had a law making it illegal to have sexual relations with a patient; Mrs. Lawrence could therefore bring criminal charges against Dr. Oldham. She could also file a malpractice suit against him, thus bringing civil charges. She could also report him to the state medical licensing board, which could temporarily or permanently take away his medical license. She could also report him to the local APA District Branch Ethics Committee, which could temporarily or permanently expel him from the American Psychiatric Association. If he were expelled this would become public knowledge since it would be reported in the *Psychiatric News,* an official organ of the APA. In addition, the psychiatrist's name would be turned over by the District Branch Ethics Committee to the state licensing board, which could then take action itself even if Mrs. Lawrence had not gone to them directly.

Finally, she could continue to choose to do nothing. If she chose the latter course, she could change her mind in the future with respect to some of the options. For example, there is no statute of limitations with regard to APA ethics complaints; she would be free to bring a complaint at any time in the future. However, there was in their state a three year statute of limitations for malpractice actions; if she waited longer than that she could no longer pursue that option.

Mrs. Lawrence told Dr. Casey that above all else she did not wish to risk public exposure; therefore, she rejected the first three options. She asked to be given more detail about the District Branch Ethics Committee. He assured her that the Committee, of which he had once been a member, operated under the strictest confidentiality and that no matter what action they might ultimately take, her name would never appear publicly. She finally did lodge a complaint with the District Branch, which resulted, after a careful investigation, in Dr. Oldham's being expelled for life from the American Psychiatric Association. Mrs. Lawrence never did exercise any of her other options.

Discussion

All residents should be aware from the beginning of their training of the variety and the seriousness of the sanctions that can be imposed on psychiatrists who become sexually involved with their patients. The above patient pursued only one option. She could have pursued all four. It would be theoretically possible for a psychiatrist to be expelled for life from the APA, to lose his license to practice medicine, to have a several hundred thousand dollar civil damage penalty lodged against him (which his insurance company might not be willing to pay), and to be guilty of criminal charges as well. In addition, he would probably have caused severe damage to his patient. It is a heavy price to pay for a brief sexual relationship.

The method of using an experienced psychiatrist, not involved with the patient's therapy, as a consultant is discussed in more detail in Stone (1984).

Discussion Questions

1. Suppose Mrs. Lawrence had continued to refuse to pursue any course of action and did not wish Dr. Youngfield to do so either. Would it be ethically justified for Dr. Youngfield to call Dr. Oldham, off-the-record, identify himself, tell Dr. Oldham that a patient he could not name had reported that she had had a sexual relationship with Dr. Oldham, encourage him to seek therapy, and warn him never to repeat his action in the future?
2. Again, suppose Mrs. Lawrence wished no action to be taken. Would it be ethically justifiable for Dr. Youngfield to write to the District Branch Ethics Committee anonymously and alert them to the fact that Dr. Oldham had allegedly had sexual relations with a patient, so that in the event of a future complaint against Dr. Oldham the District Branch would be aware he was probably a repeat offender?

References

Gartrell, N., Herman, J., Olarte, O., et al. (1986). Psychiatrist-patient sexual contact: Results of a national survey, I: Prevalence. *American Journal of Psychiatry, 143,* 1126–1131.

Stone, A. A. (1984). *Law, psychiatry, and morality* (pp. 191–216). Washington, DC: American Psychiatric Association Press.

American Psychiatric Association Subcommittee on the Education of Psychiatrists on Ethical Issues. (1986). *Ethical concerns about sexual involvement between psychiatrists and patients* [Film]. Washington, DC: American Psychiatric Association.

6

CONFIDENTIALITY; DOUBLE-AGENTRY

CASE 15. BREACHING CONFIDENTIALITY

Three months ago, a 26-year-old married man, Mr. McCoy, began outpatient treatment for what appeared to be panic attacks and growing agoraphobia. He had been bothered by episodic anxiety and depression throughout most of his adult life, but this was the first time that he had sought professional treatment. He had been married for one year and said the marriage was the best thing that had ever happened to him. He was symptom free until six months into the marriage, when he began having panic attacks whenever he traveled from his suburban home into the city. These worsened to the point that he refused to go into the city; he was now in danger of losing his job, which required periodic trips there.

His psychiatrist, Dr. Liatris, began a program of combined pharmacotherapy and psychotherapy. With imipramine and once-weekly insight-oriented psychotherapy his symptoms largely resolved. Furthermore, important information about the source of his anxiety was gradually revealed. He acknowledged that he was bisexual prior to his marriage. His occasional homosexual encounters consisted of anonymous sex in gay bars and bath houses. These occurred infrequently and generally in the context of a deepening depression, which they seemed to help resolve. His homosexual desires were generally ego-dystonic; he struggled to resist them, but with only limited success. The liaisons that did occur acquired a dissociative quality that frightened him. He came to realize during therapy that one motivation for getting married was to try to better control his homosexual desires, which he did not see as morally wrong but as seriously dangerous to his physical health.

Mr. McCoy promised himself not to engage in any further homosexual activity after he was married. For the first six months he was successful. Then he nearly picked up a man one night after he was passed over for a long sought-after promotion. His confidence about being able to continue to resist his homosexual impulses was sorely shaken and he began to have panic attacks whenever he was in the section of the city where he used to meet men. He had not engaged in any homosexual activity since his marriage and did not want his wife informed about his past life. Soon after learning of Mr. McCoy's past homosexual activity, Dr. Liatris raised the issue of AIDS and whether Mrs. McCoy might now be in some danger. Mr. McCoy acknowledged the danger but at first refused to be tested, arguing that he had no symptoms, was sure he didn't have the virus, and that neither he nor his wife could bear the news if he did test positively.

Dr. Liatris was unsure what to do. He felt the patient's wife might be in some danger, but hesitated to breach confidentiality without having any more information than was available. He decided to continue therapy for a few sessions, though that might slightly increase Mrs. McCoy's risk, in order to explore the reasons behind the patient's fear and denial. During the next session, Mr. McCoy mentioned that he and his wife wanted to have children and were currently trying to conceive. When Dr. Liatris informed him of the possible AIDS risk to any future child, he seemed startled. He had not realized he was placing a possible child at risk. With obviously increased anxiety, he consented to testing and stated that he would inform his wife if he should be HIV+.

Serologic testing and confirmation were positive. Mr. McCoy experienced a significant exacerbation of anxiety, including several episodes of derealization and depersonalization that made him fear he was "losing my mind." He now refused to tell his wife, believing that telling her would cause him to lose both his wife and his sanity, the only things he had left. Should Dr. Liatris inform Mrs. McCoy?

Discussion

The rule against breaching confidentiality is a strong one in medical practice. Patients need to know that almost anything they reveal to a physician will go no further, and nowhere is the need for confidentiality greater than in psychiatric practice. Patients in psychotherapy must be able to trust that they can speak openly about their experiences and their feelings without fear that the therapist will tell others what they have said.

It is part of a physician's duty to keep confidences. To breach confidentiality is to violate a moral rule with respect to a patient. However, the duty to keep confidences, strong as it is, is not absolute. Moral rules are universal—they apply at all times—but no moral rule is absolute. Even killing can, rarely, be ethically justified, as in self-defense, but the burden of proof is always on the person who violates a moral rule to justify ethically its violation. The criteria for a justified moral rule violation are similar to the criteria given above for a justified paternalistic action. That is not surprising: Paternalistic actions always involve moral rule violations and for this reason require ethical justification. That is, it must be true that violating the moral rule, despite the harm that would result from always violating the rule in cases of this kind, would probably prevent sufficient harm that some rational persons would agree that violations should occur in cases of this kind.

Should a physician breach confidentiality when his patient is HIV+ and the patient's wife has no reason to suspect her husband's sero-positivity? Most would say yes, including the Council on Ethical and Judicial Affairs of the American Medical Association (1988). The breach would certainly cause harm to the patient: distress that his wife will now know of his bisexuality and his HIV status, and the resultant turmoil that will cause in his marriage. There is another kind of harm that would result. Since it would become generally known that physicians feel ethically justified in breaching confidentiality in certain, albeit extreme, kinds of cases, there might be some weakening of the trust that patients put in physicians to keep any kind of confidence. But the harm that the breach may prevent is great: the wife's infection with a fatal disease.

How likely is it that she may become infected, if she is not already? Precise figures are not known. Some observers have estimated that the risk of HIV transmission from a single act of unprotected vaginal intercourse is on the order of 1 in 500 (Hearst & Hulley, 1988). Since the patient's wife does not know that her husband has engaged in homosexual encounters, she has no reason to believe that unprotected intercourse poses any danger to her of contracting AIDS.

If the 1 in 500 figure is correct, and if the couple engages in unprotected vaginal intercourse twice weekly, then the wife has a roughly 20% chance per year of becoming infected with a disease that will probably be fatal. To most observers, the harm caused by the breach is so much less than the harm possibly prevented that the breach seems justified. That is, most persons would be willing to make a general exception to the rule against breaking confidences: break them in those, but only in those, situations where there is a high probability that evil(s) of great magnitude may be prevented. (The fact that this couple was trying to have children makes the breach even more strongly justified, because of the risk, probably about 50%, that, should his wife become infected, any child born from their union would be HIV+.)

The ethical reasoning underlying this case is similar to that underlying other duty-to-warn cases. For example, psychiatrists have an ethical duty, and in most jurisdictions a legal duty as well, to warn (or otherwise protect) potential victims who may be in danger from patients under their care, even when they must breach confidentiality to do so. A similar duty exists in involuntary hospitalization cases: If the psychiatrist feels that his mentally ill patient poses a significant threat to himself or to others, the patient must be hospitalized, against his wishes if necessary. In the process of documenting in writing and later testifying in court about the need for hospitalization, the psychiatrist may need to divulge information that ordinarily would be confidential. The ethical reasoning justifying the breach in all of these kinds of cases is similar: Though the breach causes harm, both to the individual patient toward whom it is committed, and to all present and future patients because there is some weakening of the trust that may be placed in psychiatrists never to reveal private information, these harms are believed to be out-weighed by the possible prevention of serious harm to particular individuals.

In both the duty-to-warn and the involuntary hospitalization kinds of cases, one persistent problem has been the lack of knowledge, even in cohorts of patients who are believed to be above average in level of dangerousness (for example, those who are depressed, impulsive, and have a means available of killing themselves) about how frequently harmful behavior would in fact occur without psychiatric intervention. Ethical judgments should depend on data, in particular on estimates of the probability of harms pursuant to different courses of action. Our judgment about the ethical justifiability of detaining a patient, as discussed above, might change if we knew there was a 1% versus a 25% chance that patients in this patient's category would seriously harm themselves if they were not detained. It is interesting that in duty-to-warn of HIV+ cases we do have more precise estimates available (for example, approximately a 20% per year chance of transmitting a fatal disease to a regular sexual partner) against which to test and calibrate our moral intuitions.

Discussion Questions

1. If you agree that in the above case it is morally justified to breach confidentiality and inform Mr. McCoy's unsuspecting wife, how would you propose Dr. Liatris go about conveying that information to her?

2. How far would you extend the judgment that a breach is ethically justifiable? Suppose Mr. McCoy had several male friends with whom he had occasional but regular sexual contact; would you inform them of his HIV+ status?

3. Do you think Dr. Liatris should have informed Mr. McCoy at the outset that in the event the HIV testing turned out to be

positive, he believed that Mrs. McCoy needed to be informed, even if Mr. McCoy were to change his mind and no longer wish to tell her? If your answer is yes, how would you respond to the argument that your giving this information to Mr. McCoy might cause him to obtain anonymous HIV testing, which is generally available, to prevent Dr. Liatris from ever knowing his HIV status? That is, if it is ethically justifiable to breach confidentiality in the case as outlined, would it also be ethically justifiable, to protect Mrs. McCoy, not to tell Mr. McCoy about one's intentions of informing her if the testing is positive, no matter what Mr. McCoy wishes?

References

American Psychiatric Association. (1987). Guidelines on confidentiality. *American Journal of Psychiatry, 144,* 1522–1526.

Council on Ethical and Judicial Affairs. (1988). Ethical issues involved in the growing AIDS crisis. *Journal of the American Medical Association, 259,* 1360–1361.

Hearst, N., & Hulley, S. B. (1988). Preventing the heterosexual spread of AIDS. Are we giving our patients the best advice? *Journal of the American Medical Association, 259,* 2428–2432.

CASE 16. REPORTING CHILD ABUSE

Dr. Levine had been treating Mrs. Brown, the wife of a successful local politician, for two years. Therapy focused on Mrs. Brown's inability to accomplish certain goals, in particular her inability to finish her doctoral dissertation. Four months ago Mrs. Brown gave birth to a healthy baby boy. She resumed psychotherapy one month after delivery.

Late one afternoon Dr. Levine received a call from Mr. Brown. Mrs. Brown had confided to her husband that earlier that afternoon she had experienced thoughts of wanting to kill her son. She had been bathing him, and when he would not stop crying, she shook him very hard, then held his head under water in the tub. After a few seconds she became startled by what she was doing, and brought the child above water and comforted him.

Dr. Levine met with the Browns immediately. Mrs. Brown explained that she was frightened and ashamed of her behavior. She claimed that never before had she had the slightest impulse to hurt her child. She denied hallucinations, feelings of depression or anger, and reported that things seemed to be going well at home. Her husband agreed.

Dr. Levine and the Browns agreed that Mrs. Brown should not be left alone with the child in the near future. Mr. Brown said that he could arrange time off to care for the infant. Mrs. Brown promised to tell her husband and Dr. Levine immediately if she experienced any further impulses to harm the child.

One week later Dr. Levine saw the Browns again. Everything appeared to be going well. Mrs. Brown appeared neither psychotic nor depressed. Again, she described feeling frightened and ashamed about her previous actions, but had experienced no impulses whatsoever to hurt her child. She praised her husband's willingness to help out but denied feeling overwhelmed or out of control in any way. At the end of the session, all agreed that Mrs. Brown could resume care of the infant. She promised to call her husband or Dr. Levine immediately if anything changed.

Dr. Levine remained puzzled by this incident. Why, he wondered, did a woman with no serious past psychopathology, and no previous thoughts of wanting to hurt her infant, suddenly go as far as she did toward hurting him? He knew that what she had done represented child abuse and that technically he should report it, but he decided not to do so because it might damage their psychotherapeutic relationship. Also, given her husband's public job, he felt that reporting might ultimately cause the family more harm than good. He did make a mental note to call the Browns in four or five days to see how matters were progressing. Two days later Dr. Levine received a call from Mr. Brown: Mrs. Brown had been found sitting on her bed, her fatally drowned infant at her side, saying, "I couldn't help doing it."

Discussion

Laws requiring the reporting of actual or suspected child abuse are written strictly in most states: Both must always be reported by health care workers to the appropriate child protective services. While some medical and legal commentators believe physicians have a slight degree of discretion about whether to report, most would claim that in this case, where a clear incident of abuse had occurred, Dr. Levine had no discretion about reporting. The harm that reporting might do to the father or the family should not have been, from the law's point of view, a consideration; neither should Dr. Levine's clinical judgment that the child was not at present in any danger of harm. The laws may be written as they are because of the legislatures' judgments that the harm to children that may be caused by families is so great, and so important to avoid, that it is best to err on the side of overreporting.

If Dr. Levine had reported an actual instance of abuse of this kind, child protective services in many locales would have removed the child from Mrs. Brown's care for a period of time, and the child's death might have been averted. However, what makes Dr. Levine's failure to report unethical, most would argue, is not that his clinical judgment was incorrect (cf. Case 9), but that he did not have adequate justification for not obeying the applicable law. His not reporting would have been unethical even if the Brown baby had never sustained any future harm from his mother.

Discussion Questions

1. Did Dr. Levine have reasonable assurance that Mrs. Brown would not harm her baby? How do you view Mrs. Brown's assertion that she had never had the slightest impulse to harm her child?

2. Do you agree with the claim that all "suspected" instances of child abuse should be reported? Suppose you interview a family and you have only a mild suspicion that abuse may exist. Should you have discretion about reporting? What should you do?

3. What are the laws about reporting actual and suspected child abuse in your state? As the above case illustrates, it is not only child psychiatrists who need to be familiar with reporting requirements.

CASE 17. DOUBLE AGENTRY: CONFLICTS WITH THE PATIENT'S BEST INTERESTS

Dr. Cardoba was a 34-year-old psychiatrist who had been trained at a major university medical center. She recently opened her practice in a medium-sized mid-western city. A new psychiatric hospital had begun admitting patients in her section of the city. She was visited by a representative of that hospital and invited to consider admitting some of her patients there. The representative emphasized the many attractive features of the new clinical setting, and also described some financial incentives the hospital had in place for physicians who admitted there. Depending on the number of bed-days per year her patients were in the hospital, she would receive a proportionate year-end bonus based on the hospital's profit for the year. High-volume users would also be rewarded by receiving preferential referrals to their outpatient practice from the hospital.

Dr. Cardoba promised to consider the offer. The representative left behind some sophisticated and attractive promotional material. As Dr. Cardoba reflected on the offer she was of two minds. The new hospital already had a good reputation, it was conveniently located for the majority of her patients, and the financial incentives being offered were extremely attractive. At the same time she was suspicious about the hospital's unabashed emphasis on length of stay, money, and profit. Was there some way in which such an institution might compromise her standards of good psychiatric practice?

Discussion

There is little doubt that a variety of changes in the way in which health care is being delivered and reimbursed is altering the complexion of American psychiatric practice. (An excellent summary of some of these changes and their implication for psychiatric practice may be found in Ethics Committee, 1988). These changes take many forms: the growth of private psychiatric hospitals; the creation of new structures for delivering health care, like Health Maintenance Organizations (HMOs) or

Preferred Provider Organizations; and the creation of new kinds of financial incentives for physicians, incentives which sometimes reward a physician for using a clinical service less, sometimes for using it more.

Most of these new arrangements for delivering psychiatric care have important ethical aspects. One ethical problem many of them share is that they place the psychiatrist in a possible double-agentry position. That is, the psychiatrist, while she continues to be the agent for the patient's best interests, also has some incentive to satisfy interests that may compete with the patient's.

The arrangement Dr. Cardoba is considering is like that. Imagine that she is deciding whether to hospitalize a patient, or whether to extend the hospital stay of a patient once he is admitted. What was best for the patient would certainly influence her, but she would also be aware that every time she opted for increased hospital use she would be increasing her year-end bonus, and making it more likely that she would receive potentially lucrative outpatient referrals from the hospital. Even if she were not venal—she would never hospitalize anyone, say, *just* to make money—would she tilt in the direction of hospitalization in borderline cases? When her own personal financial interests conflict with what would be best for a patient, the opportunity for self-deception is present even when she tries to be as objective as possible.

Some of the new financial arrangements in medicine do not reward the high use of services, but rather the low. This is true of many prepaid plans, like HMOs, where there is a finite pool of money paid into the plan each year by subscribers. Clinical services are paid for out of these funds. At the end of each year there is more money left in the pool if clinical services have been used less, and this leftover money may be divided among physicians participating in the HMO. Thus, not to order a test of thyroid function on a depressed patient, to use drug treatment rather than psychotherapy, to have mental health treatment carried out by lower-paid rather than higher-paid mental health professionals—all of these save money, money which may in part be retained by the same physicians who make these clinical decisions. Many of these individual decisions may be in a patient's best interests, but the possibility of subjective bias seems strong and should be acknowledged and addressed.

Problems with double-agentry are not new to psychiatry. Psychiatrists who work for courts, prison, colleges, and in the military are often in a position where they have a responsibility to their patients but some responsibility also to the institutions that employ them, and instances of conflict between the two can arise. But in these cases, the psychiatrist's own personal interests are usually not at stake, or at least not in as compelling a way, as can be true in the new reimbursement schemes.

It is true that even traditional fee-for-service medicine has potential double-agentry problems, for example, whether to increase the frequency or duration of psychotherapy with a patient with an excellent bill-paying record. What is different about the new financial arrangements is the pervasiveness of the double-agentry, where the majority of the clinician's decisions may redound on her own financial interests. In fee-for-service medicine, although physicians' decisions commonly have financial implications, it is often others (hospitals, clinical laboratories) who stand to profit or not, and not the physician directly herself.

We do not mean to impugn out-of-hand these new arrangements for delivering mental health care. There is little evidence yet about whether they result in better, worse, or even discriminably different care for patients. What does seem necessary, at a minimum, is that practitioners realize the extent of the double-agentry problem and, just as importantly, that patients be informed of the nature of these reimbursement schemes.

The necessity for disclosure to patients is a part of the general ethical requirements of valid consent. Patients should be given the opportunity to learn the nature of any arrangement they enter before they consent to participate. If an HMO will pay for no more than four or six therapy sessions per year, patients need to know that before enrolling. If, at the time of recommending antidepressant medication, the psychiatrist realizes that if this were a private patient, she would strongly recommend psychotherapy as well in order to achieve an optimal result, the patient should be told that. If Dr. Cardoba stands to profit every time she admits a patient to the new private hospital, patients to whom she recommends admission should know that, perhaps in a brochure they are given at the time she initially sees them.

In many or most cases, patients may not do anything differently after they have been given the facts about such arrangements. However, disclosure may motivate the patient, if he desires and if he can afford it, to go outside the system and purchase additional care, or obtain a second opinion. It also makes it clear to the patient that his doctor is an honest person. In our experience full disclosure does not harm and often strengthens the doctor-patient relationship.

Dr. Cardoba accepted the offer to join the admitting staff of the new hospital. However, after she had been admitting patients there for several months she discovered several things that led her to resign and to use other local hospitals for her patients. She learned that there was not full medical control over admissions, and that substantial veto power was given to administrative personnel who screened patients for their ability to pay and their credit rating. The hospital also began actively to discourage her from admitting any of her patients elsewhere. The final straw came when she was called in by an administrator, was told that the average length-of-stay for patients at the hospital was 28 days but that she was discharging after an average of only 21 days, and was encouraged in strong terms to increase her average.

Discussion Questions

1. By no means do all private psychiatric hospitals pressure their staffs the way in which Dr. Cardoba was pressured. How could she have tried to learn in advance some of the hospital's policies which she later found disturbing? Make up a list of questions which a psychiatrist could ask ahead of time to try to ferret out reimbursement policies which are ethically problematic.

2. If a psychiatrist works for an HMO, she may be asked to agree to see patients for no more than, say, five times a year. Is it ethical for a psychiatrist to enter into such an agreement, knowing that inevitably some patients whom she sees will need more extensive care than that?

3. It is not only private hospitals that can raise problems of double-agentry for the psychiatrist. What double-agentry problems might be present in a community mental health center? In a university student mental health center?

References

Dougherty, C. J. (1988). Mind, money, and morality: Ethical dimensions of economic change in American psychiatry. *Hastings Center Report, 18,* 15–20.

Ethics Committee of the American Psychiatric Association. (1988). New mental health economics and the impact on the ethics of practice: A report of the Hastings Center Conference on psychiatric ethics and new economics. *Ethics Newsletter, April-May,* 1–7.

Webb, W. L. (1989). Ethical psychiatric practice in a new economic climate. *Psychiatric Annals, 19,* 443–447.

7

SUMMARY AND REVIEW OF BASIC ETHICAL CONCEPTS

The preceding cases have all involved the application to clinical situations of concepts and decision-making procedures derived from moral philosophy. After each case, conceptual material was introduced which seemed most relevant to the facts at hand. In this final chapter we summarize and elaborate some parts of the conceptual material previously introduced. Though the chapter is inevitably somewhat redundant, it seems useful to have a more integrated account available.

Valid Consent or Refusal

The concept of valid consent or refusal is probably the most basic of all concepts in medical ethics. It figured prominently in many of the preceding cases. A great many other issues in medical ethics are linked closely to it. It is commonly held, both ethically and legally, that in order for a patient's consent or refusal to be valid, three criteria must be met: the patient must receive *adequate information* about the test, treatment or procedure that is being suggested; *no coercion* can be used in obtaining the consent; and the patient must be *fully competent* to consent or refuse. These concepts were defined briefly in Case 1; we give a fuller account here.

Adequate Information. How much information must be given to satisfy the criterion of adequacy? A simple general answer is that any information should be given that a rational person would want to know before making a decision to consent or refuse. At the minimum, a rational person would want to know the significant harms and benefits that are possibly or probably associated with a suggested treatment, with any rational alternative treatments, and with no treatment at all.

The language in which most patients want harms and benefits to be expressed is in terms of the basic harms that will likely be caused, prevented, or ameliorated by various courses of action. The harms which concern rational persons are: death; pain (physical or mental); various disabilities; and loss of freedom, opportunity or pleasure. Technical language need not be used in giving explanations. Few patients, for example, have any interest in current speculation about the important sites of dopamine blockade in the central nervous system, or how that blockade might reverse certain kinds of psychotic symptoms. They are concerned, however, with the probability that a drug will make them feel less psychic pain, and with the concomitant risk that the same drug might cause painful spasms of the muscles.

How probable must it be that a harm may occur in conjunction with a treatment before a patient should be told about it? That is a joint function of the severity of the harm and the likelihood of its occurrence. Any nontrivial risk of death (say, 1 in 10,000 or more) should be told: Death is such a serious harm that rational persons are always concerned with any nontrivial risk that it might occur. Less serious harms of a low probability need not be told, for example, tinnitus caused by heterocyclic antidepressants. The criterion for disclosure should always be: Would a rational person want to know this risk before making an informed decision? This is the test dictated not only by ethics but increasingly by the courts in cases where the completeness of disclosure has been challenged in malpractice actions. The basic notion was well-expressed by one judge (*Canterbury v. Spence,* 1972): "The patient's right of self-decision shapes the boundaries of the duty to disclose."

When rare but serious side effects are associated with a treatment, it is often sufficient to tell patients just that—that there are rare but serious side effects—and to describe them only if the patient requests it. The agranulocytosis that occurs rarely after heterocyclic therapy probably falls in this category.

Patients should be told about any rational alternatives that exist for treatment of their disorder other than the alternative being suggested. One useful test of whether such alternatives exist is to ask oneself whether some other competent psychiatrist might suggest some other treatment in the situation at hand. Thus, to suggest only intensive psychotherapy to a patient with a mild to moderate depression, when one knows that other psychiatrists would also use drug therapy, is to give the patient insufficient information about possible treatments. Many psychiatrists believe that combined treatment is beneficial: Drugs may shorten the duration of depression without diminishing the usefulness of on-going psychotherapy. The patient needs to know about both treatment possibilities, as well as why his psychiatrist is recommending psychotherapy alone, before he can decide for himself which he prefers.

Finally, patients should be told about what is apt to happen to them in the absence of any treatment. Some reactive psychological disorders, for example, have a reasonably good chance of improving simply with the passage of time. Before undertaking a lengthy or an expensive trial of one or more treatments, that would be important information for patients to know. Other disorders, especially emergent psychotic ones, are less apt to improve on their own.

Absence of Coercion. Consent is not valid if coercion has been used in obtaining it. "Coercion" is a term sometimes given a broad definition, but a narrow one is intended here. "Coercion" refers to the use of such powerful negative incentives (for example, threat of severe pain or significant deprivation of freedom) that it would be unreasonable to expect a person to resist them. Thus, a psychiatrist uses coercion if she threatens a suicidal patient with detainment in a state hospital if he does not continue his "voluntary" treatment elsewhere. It is sometimes morally justifiable (and legally permitted) to coerce patients into treatment, but of course the treatment is not being carried out with the patient's voluntary consent; thus, the burden of proof is on the psychiatrist to furnish explicit arguments about why the coercion is ethically justified.

Having said what "coercion" is, it is just as important to say what it is not. It is not coercive to recommend a treatment strongly, or even to argue pointedly for it. Most patients want to know what treatment their doctor thinks is best. Also, most persons know their initial decisions about treatment may be overly influenced by emotional reactions that may change upon reflection, and they do not mind a degree of challenge. What is important is for the psychiatrist to be open and objective in describing the available alternative treatments and to be specific about why she is particularly recommending one, if she is. The patient should know throughout that after the discussion about treatments is over, the final decision will be his alone to make, and that the doctor will not abandon or psychologically punish him if he chooses contrary to her recommendation.

Patient Competence. In order for consent to be valid, patients must be fully competent to consent to or refuse treatment. What is meant by "competence"? This is a somewhat complex matter, but it is important for psychiatrists to be clear in their understanding and use of this term. The assessment of competence is widely regarded as an activity in which psychiatrists are particularly skilled, and they commonly receive requests from the courts and from their medical and surgical colleagues to assess a patient's competence.

Competence is best regarded not as a global characteristic of patients, so that each patient must be classified as either totally competent or totally incompetent. It is more precise and accurate to regard competence as tied to some specific activity. Thus, a patient may be quite competent to feed himself or dress himself, but be incompetent to perform some abstract intellectual task. Similarly, a patient may be competent to perform some intellectual tasks but not others, for example, he may be able to make a simple treatment decision, but not a more complex one.

In order to decide whether a patient is competent to perform an activity, it is first necessary, whenever possible, to establish explicit criteria which, if satisfied, will establish competence in that activity. For example, in many jurisdictions someone is judged legally competent to make a will if the following criteria are satisfied: She must know what her assets are; know who her natural heirs are (who would inherit her goods in the absence of a will); and know, at the pertinent time, that she is making out a will. If these criteria are satisfied, the will has been made out competently and cannot be successfully challenged on the grounds of the competency of its maker.

What concerns us here are the criteria that should be used to judge whether a patient is competent to consent to or refuse treatment. That is not the only kind of competency that psychiatrists are asked to evaluate; competency to stand trial, competency to manage one's financial affairs, even "competency to be executed" are others. We will not discuss other species of competency here, except to suggest that each of them is best evaluated by first establishing explicit criteria relevant to the ability at hand.

We believe the relevant criterion for assessing competence to consent to or refuse treatment is *the degree to which the patient is able to understand and appreciate the information that is conveyed during an adequate consent process.* This is the most widely used criterion for competence to consent or refuse in both medical ethics and in health law. It is necessary to include both understanding and appreciation in the criterion, because there are occasional patients who understand the relevant information but do not appreciate that it applies to them, for example, a man who suffers from the delusion that he is Superman and that no harm can befall him. He might understand the possible harms and benefits of a treatment quite well, but also believe that while they might occur to other people they could not occur to him because he is Superman.

Note that competence is a set of cognitive abilities that patients do or do not have. Competence is not related to a patient's actual decision, that is, whether he consents or refuses. This is because the whole point of establishing whether a patient is competent is to allow competent patients, almost always, to make any treatment decision they wish. If a patient's actual decision (i.e., whether he consents or refuses) were ever the criterion of competence, one would be saying that some decisions, no matter how well the patient understands and appreciates the relevant information, render him incompetent. That would vitiate the whole point of the concept of competence. It is important to evaluate the patient's actual treatment decision, and we will suggest below doing so in terms of whether it is rational or irrational, but that is a different matter from evaluating the competence of the patient to make it.*

Competence and rationality are different concepts. They do not even apply to the same kind of thing. One can make no certain conclusion about a patient's degree of competence from knowing her actual decision. Thus, if a patient consents to treatment, which would nearly always be a rational decision, it does not necessarily follow that the patient is competent to consent to treatment. Similarly, if a patient refuses treatment, and that refusal is irrational, it does not necessarily follow that the patient is not competent to refuse treatment.

Using the criterion of a patient's degree of ability to understand and appreciate the relevant information, patients may be divided into three categories: some are incompetent, some are partially competent, and some are fully competent to consent or refuse.

It is necessary to have a three-fold classification of competence in order to describe adequately the phenomena of clinical practice. Some patients, the incompetent, cannot consent or refuse, and it seems important to divide those who can and do consent or refuse into two categories: those who adequately understand and appreciate the information relevant to their decisions and those who do not. Each of these categories of patients should be and in fact is treated differently in clinical practice.

---

*A few theorists believe that the rationality of the patient's decision should enter into the evaluation of the patient's competence (see Drane, 1985; Buchanan & Brock, 1986). Others believe doing so leads to harmful conceptual confusion (Culver & Gert, unpublished manuscript).

Incompetent patients are unable to consent or refuse at all. They may be either comatose and completely unaware of their surroundings, or they may have limited cognitive abilities but still be unable to understand the consent process. If one does suggest a treatment, the patient either cannot answer or answers in some random fashion. These patients have no or essentially no degree of understanding or appreciation. Many medical and surgical patients are transiently or permanently incompetent, but psychiatric patients may be as well.

Partially competent patients understand that they are being asked to consent or refuse, and they do consistently consent or refuse, but they lack the ability to understand and appreciate adequately the information given to them during the consent process. They may be described as giving a simple consent or refusal, but not a valid consent or refusal. This category of patients is seen frequently in medical practice, especially among patients suffering from a delirium. Psychiatric patients are not uncommonly only partially competent. This may be because of a delirium, because of a degree of dementia, or because of psychiatric symptoms that affect the patient's ability to understand and appreciate information.

The overwhelming majority of patients are *fully competent.* They understand the information given to them during the consent process, and they appreciate that it applies to them at this point in time. Whether one thinks the decision they have made is wise or foolish—even if one would label it as seriously irrational—they are fully competent to have made it.

Competence is a legal term as well as a clinical concept. Some say it is only or primarily a legal term but that seems mistaken. It is true that only a court can declare someone "legally incompetent." It is also true that some courts prefer that a psychiatrist testifying at a competence hearing avoid using the term "competence" itself during the hearing, but instead confine her expert remarks to describing such matters as the patient's ability to understand and appreciate information, thus allowing the court to make the final judgment about competence. However, in the ordinary clinical setting, it is psychiatrists who are asked to appraise competence, and in most of these cases, unless a psychiatrist believes a patient is incompetent, the case would never reach the court in the first place. Thus, even if one were concerned only with the courts, psychiatrists would need to understand the concept thoroughly and know when the legal threshold of incompetence had been reached, or nearly reached.

Competence is also more than a legal concept in the sense that judgments about patients' competence influence the clinical behavior of physicians constantly, and it is appropriate that they do so. For example, as patients with fatal chronic illnesses come nearer to death, it frequently happens that they become no longer competent to make decisions about continuation of their life-support systems. Unless the patient's advance wishes are sufficiently clearly known, physicians at some point usually need to rely on family members' proxy decisions, or on a Durable Power of Attorney for Health Care. However, as long as the patient is competent, it is his wishes that should be determinative. Thus, a judgment needs to be made about when competence is lost. Sometimes this is clear, sometimes not. It is helpful, when unsure, to have a clear conception of competence to guide one's judgments. (See Case 3 above.)

These kinds of clinical situations are common. If the attending physician understands the concept of competence, a psychiatrist rarely needs to become involved, let alone a court. Psychiatrists, if they understand the concept of competence, are helpful in difficult cases. Courts need to become involved only rarely, usually in cases where there is a significant conflict between two or more parties. The clinical appraisal of competence is so common (though physicians sometimes do not label what they are doing as such) that it is fortunate that courts hardly ever need be involved; they would be glutted with cases if they heard more than the smallest fraction.

Rationality and Irrationality

Competence and rationality are not synonyms, although sometimes they are loosely used as such. Patients who are partially or fully competent to consent or refuse may make treatment decisions that are either rational or irrational. A patient's competence may be determined during the consent process, whereas the rationality of his decision is determined by his actual consent or refusal. Thus, the two concepts are conceptually independent, though they are probably empirically related: Seriously irrational treatment refusals are commonly made by patients who are only partially competent, but they may be made by patients who are fully competent.

What is an irrational decision or action? A definition of the concept was given in Case 6 and will be briefly repeated here. *A decision or action is irrational if its foreseeable results are that the person will suffer harms without an adequate reason.* What is an "adequate reason"?

A *reason* is a conscious belief that one's decision or action will help oneself (or someone else) avoid or relieve some harm or gain some good. Thus, if I believe that by enduring some pain (for example, suffering the mild side effects associated with an antidepressant drug) I have a high probability of ameliorating some other pain (for example, mental depression), that belief is a reason for enduring the first pain.

Although there can be reasons for any kind of action, we talk of adequate reasons only when the action contemplated would be irrational if there were no reason for doing it. A reason is an *adequate reason* when some rational persons would agree that the harms likely to be avoided (or the goods gained) by suffering the harms of the contemplated act compensate for the harms caused by that act.

Thus, not all reasons are adequate reasons. Recall the example of having a leg amputated in order to eliminate the mild pain caused by a small plantar wart. No rational person would agree that the harms incurred by losing a leg are compensated for by the elimination of the mild pain from a wart. Having the leg amputated, however, to try to stop the spread of an osteogenic sarcoma in the tibia would count as an adequate reason and would therefore be a rational treatment decision. Thus, the effect of having an adequate reason is to turn an otherwise irrational action or decision into a rational one.

It is rarely irrational for a patient to consent to a treatment suggested by a competent physician. That is because competent physicians rarely suggest irrational treatments. An irrational treatment is one from which a patient, on balance, has a great deal more to lose than to gain, and competent physicians should not suggest such a course of action.

However, even though a suggested treatment is rational, it is often quite rational for a patient to refuse it. A dysthymic patient, for example, may rationally refuse or consent to an extended and/or expensive course of intensive psychotherapy for his depression. There is sometimes the temptation, until one reflects on it, to think that if one alternative in a situation is rational, then other alternatives are irrational, but there are frequently multiple rational alternatives in a particular situation.

In many situations, however, it is irrational for a patient to refuse a suggested treatment. This is true of the treatment refusals of some seriously depressed patients: They have a significant chance of dying without treatment, they have no adequate reason for dying, yet they refuse treatment nonetheless. Sometimes such patients are partially incompetent, but sometimes they are fully competent. The important moral (and legal) issue which arises in this setting is: When is it justified to treat these patients against their will? Treating patients who do not wish to be treated is almost always an instance of paternalistic behavior.

Paternalistic Behavior and Its Ethical Justification

The concept of paternalistic behavior is another central concept in medical ethics, and has many applications in psychiatry. There have been several important attempts to define the notion of paternalistic behavior (see references listed at the end of Case 6). They agree in large part but differ in detail. The following definition is given by Culver and Gert (1982):

> An action is paternalistic when it satisfies four criteria:
>
> 1) it must be carried out with the intention of benefiting the subject;

2) it must involve the violation of a moral rule;
3) it must be carried out without the consent of the subject;
4) the subject must be at least partially competent, or be expected to become partially competent, to give consent. (p. 130)

As discussed in Case 6, violating a moral rule involves acting toward someone in a way that either directly inflicts a harm on the person, for example, killing, causing pain (physical or mental), disabling, or depriving of freedom or pleasure, or is the kind of action that increases the likelihood that the person will suffer one or more harms, for example, deceiving someone or breaking a promise one has made to someone. Violating a moral rule with regard to another person is always immoral if one does not have a morally adequate reason for doing so.

Thus, detaining a patient in a state hospital is essentially always a paternalistic action. It is done with the intention of benefiting the patient; it violates the moral rule against depriving someone of his or her freedom; it is clearly done without the patient's consent (or else it would not be detainment); and the patient is at least partially competent (i.e., at least competent enough to be refusing hospitalization).

Nearly all scholars agree that paternalistic behavior is unethical unless it can be ethically justified. That conclusion can be explained in terms of the above definition. Paternalistic behavior involves the violation of a moral rule and violating a moral rule is unethical unless it can be ethically justified. When is paternalistic behavior ethically justified? We will give here a brief but usable summary of one set of criteria for ethically justified paternalistic behavior; a fuller discussion with many case examples may be found in Culver and Gert (1982).

In order for it to be ethically justified to act paternalistically, for example, to treat an unwilling patient, four ethically relevant criteria must all be satisfied:

1) The harm or harms the treatment will probably avoid or ameliorate for the patient must be very great (death or serious physical disability).
2) The harm or harms imposed by the treatment must be, by comparison, very much less.

3) The patient's desire not to be treated must be seriously irrational.
4) The above three criteria all refer to characteristics of the particular case under consideration. It is necessary that they be satisfied to justify forced treatment, but it is not sufficient. It must also be the case that at least some impartial rational persons would advocate *always* allowing forced treatment in cases having the same ethically relevant characteristics described by the first three criteria. This fourth criterion forces the kind of impartiality which is a necessary component of ethical reasoning.

Using these criteria, it is sometimes true that forced psychiatric treatment is ethically justified and sometimes it is not. Case 6 is an example of ethically justified treatment (installation of an intravenous line), while in Case 7 it would not be justified to force neuroleptic medications.

Treating unwilling patients has important legal as well as moral implications. There is great theoretical uncertainty in this area of the law at present and psychiatrists need to accommodate the above (or some other) ethical analysis into whatever legal framework exists in their jurisdiction. This is not the place for a full analysis of the legal reasoning in the various right-to-refuse-treatment state and federal Supreme Court decisions. A few summary remarks might be helpful.

The courts usually emphasize competence as the one important concept in deciding whether a patient may be overruled. A competent patient may never be overruled, but an incompetent patient may be. However, many courts are vague in defining competence, or else they initially define it strictly, using an understand-and-appreciate definition, as we have above, but then loosen the definition considerably in later parts of their opinion, or in specifying future rules to be used by clinicians in deciding individual cases.* One reason the courts may move away from a strict understand-and-appreciate definition is their realization that it is sometimes morally justified to treat

*See *Rivers v. Katz* (1986) for one example of a shifting definition.

unwilling patients who are fully competent according to an understand-and-appreciate definition.

Our advice is that the clinician have available a clear set of guidelines specifying when forced treatment seems morally justifiable, and use those guidelines in whatever way is possible in his or her legal setting. It is often particularly useful to be able to give clear moral arguments in the probate court setting, where matters of forced treatment are often adjudicated, and where moral reasoning is often quite powerful.

Immorality, Incompetence and Impairment*

In Case 13, a resident was tempted to initiate a romantic or sexual relationship with a patient. If he had done so, he would have been acting immorally. Would that also mean he was impaired? Would it mean he was incompetent? It is useful to understand these three concepts and the relationships among them.

Immorality. A person acts unethically when he or she knowingly and intentionally causes harm, or acts in a way that increases the probability of causing harm, toward another person, and has no adequate ethical justification for doing so. Thus, it is unethical, without adequate justification, to break any of the moral rules discussed above: to kill, to cause pain (physical or mental), to disable, to deprive of freedom, to deceive, to cheat, to break a promise, to violate the law, or not to carry out one's professional duties.

Psychiatrists and other physicians often violate moral rules toward patients. For example, they prescribe treatments that cause pain and may even carry some risk of death; they deprive patients of freedom; or they disable patients. Usually, however, doctors do these things with their patients' valid consent, and consent almost always provides an adequate ethical justification for the harm-causing behavior. However, if a doctor cheats a

---

*This material was originally included in a slightly different form in the American Psychiatric Association's *Ethics Newsletter*, January/February 1986.

patient, or knowingly acts negligently, or has sex with a patient (which is unethical because it has a very high probability of harming the patient), the doctor has acted unethically.

Incompetence

A doctor is incompetent when she is unable to perform some professional function that someone occupying her particular position should be able to perform satisfactorily. Thus, a general surgeon who is no longer able to remove a gall bladder would be at least partially incompetent as a general surgeon, but a psychiatrist who cannot remove a gall bladder is not an incompetent psychiatrist. Incompetence is most often a result of a physical, mental or volitional disability, but it can be due simply to lack of adequate training.

An isolated mistake does not count as incompetence. For example, a psychiatrist who prescribes tricyclic antidepressants (TCAs) quite correctly 99.9% of the time but errs on one occasion (for example, writes a prescription for 50 mg TID of Trilafon instead of Tofranil) would not be considered incompetent to prescribe TCAs, though he has certainly erred seriously on this one occasion. However, it is not necessary that one err every time one attempts a kind of task to be considered incompetent. If this same psychiatrist wrote incorrect TCA prescriptions even 5% of the time, we might well say that he was incompetent to prescribe TCAs.

Impairment. A physician is impaired if he has a mental or neurological disorder that interferes on a significant number of occasions with his ability to practice. Substance abuse is a common example. There is no logical reason we could not also speak of a physician with a physical disorder that interferes with his ability to practice as impaired (for example, a surgeon who has become blind or who has had an arm amputated), but usually we simply refer to him as disabled.

Incompetence and impairment are closely related concepts. An impaired physician is always incompetent (or only partially competent) to carry out some professional task—that is part of the meaning of "impairment." Physicians can of course have mental or physical disorders that do not interfere with their ability to practice, but then we do not regard them as impaired.

Physicians who are incompetent are usually impaired, but they need not be. One reason a psychiatrist may not be able to carry out a function that would be expected of someone with his level of training is that he has been poorly trained. We might say of him that he is incompetent but not that he is impaired.

1. *Does acting unethically mean that one is incompetent?* Often, but not necessarily. For example, suppose a psychiatrist involuntarily hospitalizes a patient on a particular occasion without any ethical or legal justification, but purely for reasons of self-interest. That would be an unethical action, but need not mean that the psychiatrist is incompetent to commit patients. However, if a psychiatrist frequently acts unethically under certain circumstances (for example, frequently has or tries to have sexual relations with his patients), this may indicate that he lacks voluntary control over his behavior (for example, he cannot refrain from making sexual overtures to at least some women patients); thus, he may have a volitional disability. We could say that he is not competent (or only partially competent) to treat women patients, and also say that he is impaired, because volitional disabilities are one kind of mental disorder.

2. *Is it unethical to be incompetent?* Sometimes, but not necessarily. For an action to be unethical the psychiatrist must have known (or should have known) that his action was harmful or potentially harmful. If a psychiatrist were no longer competent to carry out some professional duties because of a slowly developing dementia, he might be unaware of his lack of ability. We would not say he was acting unethically if he were excusably ignorant about his disability. However, once he has been told about his disability, then, if he is able to understand and remember what he has been told, he is acting unethically if he continues to practice in the area of his disability. That is because it is unethical to knowingly practice inadequately.

References

Buchanan, A., & Brock, D. W. (1986). Deciding for others. *Milbank Quarterly, 64*, 17–94.

Canterbury v. Spence, 464 F.2d 772 (D.C. Cir., 1972).

Culver, C. M., & Gert, B. (1982). *Philosophy in medicine* (pp. 130–133). New York: Oxford.

Culver, C. M., & Gert, B. (unpublished manuscript). The inadequacy of incompetence.

Drane, J. F. (1985). The many faces of competency. *Hastings Center Report, 15,* 17–21.

Rivers v. Katz, 504 N.Y.S. 2d 74 (Ct. App., 1986).

THE PRINCIPLES OF MEDICAL ETHICS With Annotations Especially Applicable to Psychiatry, 1989 Edition*

In 1973, the American Psychiatric Association published the first edition of THE PRINCIPLES OF MEDICAL ETHICS WITH ANNOTATIONS ESPECIALLY APPLICABLE TO PSYCHIATRY. Subsequently, revisions were published as the Board of Trustees and the Assembly approved additional annotations. In July of 1980, the American Medical Association approved a new version of the Principles of Medical Ethics (the first revision since 1957) and the APA Ethics Committee[1] incorporated many of its annotations into the new Principles, which resulted in the 1981 edition and subsequent revisions.

FOREWORD

All physicians should practice in accordance with the medical code of ethics set forth in the Principles of Medical Ethics of the American Medical Association. An up-to-date expression and elaboration of these statements is found in the Opinions and Reports of the Council on Ethical and Judicial Affairs of the

*Reprinted with the permission of the American Psychiatric Association.

[1]The committee included Herbert Klemmer, M.D., Chairperson, Miltiades Zaphiropoulos, M.D., Ewald Busse, M.D., John R. Saunders, M.D., and Robert McDevitt, M.D. Serving as consultants to the APA Ethics Committee were J. Brand Brickman, M.D., William P. Camp, M.D., and Robert A. Moore, M.D.

American Medical Association.[2] Psychiatrists are strongly advised to be familiar with these documents.[3]

However, these general guidelines have sometimes been difficult to interpret for psychiatry, so further annotations to the basic principles are offered in this document. While psychiatrists have the same goals as all physicians, there are special ethical problems in psychiatric practice that differ in coloring and degree from ethical problems in other branches of medical practice, even though the basic principles are the same. The annotations are not designed as absolutes and will be revised from time to time so as to be applicable to current practices and problems.

Following are the AMA Principles of Medical Ethics, printed in their entirety, and then each principle printed separately along with an annotation especially applicable to psychiatry.

PRINCIPLES OF MEDICAL ETHICS, AMERICAN MEDICAL ASSOCIATION

Preamble

The medical profession has long subscribed to a body of ethical statements developed primarily for the benefit of the patient. As a member of this profession, a physician must recognize responsibility not only to patients but also to society, to other health professionals, and to self. The following Principles, adopted by the American Medical Association, are not laws but standards of conduct, which define the essentials of honorable behavior for the physician.

[2]Current Opinions of the Council on Ethical and Judicial Affairs, Chicago, American Medical Association, 1989.

[3]Chapters 8, Section 1 of the Bylaws of the American Psychiatric Association states, "All members of the American Psychiatric Association shall be bound by the ethical code of the medical profession, specifically defined in The Principles of Medical Ethics of the American Medical Association." In interpreting the APA Constitution and Bylaws, it is the opinion of the Board of Trustees that inactive status in no way removes a physician member from responsibility to abide by the Principles of Medical Ethics.

Section 1

A physician shall be dedicated to providing competent medical service with compassion and respect for human dignity.

Section 2

A physician shall deal honestly with patients and colleagues, and strive to expose those physicians deficient in character or competence, or who engage in fraud or deception.

Section 3

A physician shall respect the law and also recognize a responsibility to seek changes in those requirements which are contrary to the best interests of the patient.

Section 4

A physician shall respect the rights of patients, of colleagues, and of other health professionals, and shall safeguard patient confidences within the constraints of the law.

Section 5

A physician shall continue to study, apply, and advance scientific knowledge, make relevant information available to patients, colleagues, and the public, obtain consultation, and use the talents of other health professionals when indicated.

Section 6

A physician shall, in the provision of appropriate patient care, except in emergencies, be free to choose whom to serve, with whom to associate, and the environment in which to provide medical services.

Section 7

A physician shall recognize a responsibility to participate in activities contributing to an improved community.

PRINCIPLES WITH ANNOTATIONS

Following are each of the AMA Principles of Medical Ethics printed separately along with annotations especially applicable to psychiatry.

Preamble

The medical profession has long subscribed to a body of ethical statements developed primarily for the benefit of the patient. As a member of this profession, a physician must recognize responsibility not only to patients but also to society, to other health professionals, and to self. The following Principles, adopted by the American Medical Association, are not laws but standards of conduct, which define the essentials of honorable behavior for the physician.[4]

Section 1

A physician shall be dedicated to providing competent medical service with compassion and respect for human dignity.

1. The patient may place his/her trust in his/her psychiatrist knowing that the psychiatrist's ethics and professional responsibilities preclude him/her gratifying his/her own needs by exploiting the patient. This becomes particularly important because of the essentially private, highly personal, and sometimes intensely emotional nature of the relationship established with the psychiatrist.
2. A psychiatrist should not be a party to any type of policy that excludes, segregates, or demeans the dignity of any patient because of ethnic origin, race, sex, creed, age, socioeconomic status, or sexual orientation.
3. In accord with the requirements of law and accepted medical practice, it is ethical for a physician to submit his/her work to peer review and to the ultimate authority of the medi-

---

[4]Statements in italics are taken directly from the American Medical Association's Principles of Medical Ethics.

cal staff executive body and the hospital administration and its governing body. In case of dispute, the ethical psychiatrist has the following steps available:

a. Seek appeal from the medical staff decision to a joint conference committee, including members of the medical staff executive committee and the executive committee of the governing board. At this appeal, the ethical psychiatrist could request that outside opinions be considered
b. Appeal to the governing body itself.
c. Appeal to state agencies regulating licensure of hospitals if, in the particular state, they concern themselves with matters of professional competency and quality of care.
d. Attempt to educate colleagues through development of research projects and data and presentations at professional meetings and in professional journals.
e. Seek redress in local courts, perhaps through an enjoining injunction against the governing body.
f. Public education as carried out by an ethical psychiatrist would not utilize appeals based solely upon emotion, but would be presented in a professional way and without any potential exploitation of patients through testimonials

4. A psychiatrist should not be a participant in a legally authorized execution.

Section 2

A physician shall deal honestly with patients and colleagues, and strive to expose those physicians deficient in character or competence, or who engage in fraud or deception.

1. The requirement that the physician conduct himself/herself with propriety in his/her profession and in all the actions of his/her life is especially important in the case of the psychiatrist because the patient tends to model his/her behavior after that of his/her therapist by identification. Further, the necessary intensity of the therapeutic relationship may tend to

activate sexual and other needs and fantasies on the part of both patient and therapist, while weakening the objectivity necessary for control. Sexual activity with a patient is unethical. Sexual involvement with one's former patients generally exploits emotions deriving from treatment and therefore almost always is unethical.

2. The psychiatrist should diligently guard against exploiting information furnished by the patient and should not use the unique position of power afforded him/her by the psychotherapeutic situation to influence the patient in any way not directly relevant to the treatment goals.

3. A psychiatrist who regularly practices outside his/her area of professional competence should be considered unethical. Determination of professional competence should be made by peer review boards or other appropriate bodies.

4. Special consideration should be given to those psychiatrists who, because of mental illness, jeopardize the welfare of their patients and their own reputations and practices. It is ethical, even encouraged, for another psychiatrist to intercede in such situations.

5. Psychiatric services, like all medical services, are dispensed in the context of a contractual arrangement between the patient and the treating physician. The provisions of the contractual arrangement, which are binding on the physician as well as on the patient, should be explicitly established.

6. It is ethical for the psychiatrist to make a charge for a missed appointment when this falls within the terms of the specific contractual agreement with the patient. Charging for a missed appointment or for one not cancelled 24 hours in advance need not, in itself, be considered unethical if a patient is fully advised that the physician will make a such a charge. The practice, however, should be resorted to infrequently and always with the utmost consideration for the patient and his/her circumstances.

7. An arrangement in which a psychiatrist provides supervision or administration to other physicians or nonmedical persons for a percentage of their fees or gross income is not acceptable; this would constitute fee-splitting. In a team of

practitioners, or a multidisciplinary team, it is ethical for the psychiatrist to receive income for administration, research, education, or consultation. This should be based upon a mutually agreed upon and set fee or salary, open to renegotiation when a change in the time demand occurs. (See also Section 5, Annotations 2, 3, and 4,)

8. When a member has been found to have behaved unethically by the American Psychiatric Association or one of its constituent district branches, there should not be automatic reporting to the local authorities responsible for medical licensure, but the decision to report should be decided upon the merits of the case.[5]

Section 3

A physician shall respect the law and also recognize a responsibility to seek changes in those requirements which are contrary to the best interests of the patient.

1. It would seem self-evident that a psychiatrist who is a lawbreaker might be ethically unsuited to practice his/her profession. When such illegal activities bear directly upon his/her practice, this would obviously be the case. However, in other instances, illegal activities such as those concerning the right to protest social injustices might not bear on either the image of the psychiatrist or the ability of the specific psychiatrist to treat his/her patient ethically and well. While no committee or board could offer prior assurance that any illegal activity would not be considered unethical, it is conceivable that an individual could violate a law without being guilty of professionally unethical behavior. Physicians lose no right of citizenship on entry into the profession of medicine.

2. Where not specifically prohibited by local laws governing medical practice, the practice of acupuncture by a psychiatrist is not unethical per se. The psychiatrist should have professional competence in the use of acupuncture. Or, if he/she is

[5]However, state and/or federal law may impose reporting requirements with which district branches and the APA must comply.

supervising the use of acupuncture by nonmedical individuals, he/she should provide proper medical supervision. (See also Section 5, Annotations 3 and 4.)

Section 4

A physician shall respect the rights of patients, of colleagues, and of other health professionals, and shall safeguard patient confidences within the constraints of the law.

1. Psychiatric records, including even the identification of a person as a patient, must be protected with extreme care. Confidentiality is essential to psychiatric treatment. This is based in part on the special nature of psychiatric therapy as well as on the traditional ethical relationship between physician and patient. Growing concern regarding the civil rights of patients and the possible adverse effects of computerization, duplication equipment, and data banks makes the dissemination of confidential information an increasing hazard. Because of the sensitive and private nature of the information with which the psychiatrist deals, he/she must be circumspect in the information that he/she chooses to disclose to others about a patient. The welfare of the patient must be a continuing consideration.

2. A psychiatrist may release confidential information only with the authorization of the patient or under proper legal compulsion. The continuing duty of the psychiatrist to protect the patient includes fully appraising him/her of the connotations of waiving the privilege of privacy. This may become an issue when the patient is being investigated by a government agency, is applying for a position, or is involved in legal action. The same principles apply to the release of information concerning treatment to medical departments of government agencies, business organizations, labor unions, and insurance companies. Information gained in confidence about patients seen in student health services should not be released without the students' explicit permission.

3. Clinical and other materials used in teaching and writing must be adequately disguised in order to preserve the anonymity of the individuals involved.

4. The ethical responsibility of maintaining confidentiality holds equally for the consultations in which the patient may not have been present and in which the consultee was not a physician. In such instances, the physician consultant should alert the consultee to his/her duty of confidentiality.

5. Ethically the psychiatrist may disclose only that information which is relevant to a given situation. He/she should avoid offering speculation as fact. Sensitive information such as an individual's sexual orientation or fantasy material is usually unnecessary.

6. Psychiatrists are often asked to examine individuals for security purposes, to determine suitability for various jobs, and to determine legal competence. The psychiatrist must fully describe the nature and purpose and lack of confidentiality of the examination to the examinee at the beginning of the examination.

7. Careful judgment must be exercised by the psychiatrist in order to include, when appropriate, the parents or guardian in the treatment of a minor. At the same time, the psychiatrist must assure the minor proper confidentiality.

8. Psychiatrists at times may find it necessary, in order to protect the patient or the community from imminent danger, to reveal confidential information disclosed by the patient.

9. When the psychiatrist is ordered by the court to reveal the confidences entrusted to him/her by patients, he/she may comply or he/she may ethically hold the right to dissent within the framework of the law. When the psychiatrist is in doubt, the right of the patient to confidentiality and, by extension, to unimpaired treatment, should be given priority. The psychiatrist should reserve the right to raise the question of adequate need for disclosure. In the event that the necessity for legal disclosure is demonstrated by the court, the psychiatrist may request the right to disclosure of only that information which is relevant to the legal question at hand.

10. With regard for the person's dignity and privacy and with truly informed consent, it is ethical to present a patient to a scientific gathering, if the confidentiality of the presentation is understood and accepted by the audience.

11. It is ethical to present a patient or former patient to a public gathering or to the news media only if the patient is fully informed of enduring loss of confidentiality, is competent, and consents in writing without coercion.

12. When involved in funded research, the ethical psychiatrist will advise human subjects of the funding source, retain his/her freedom to reveal data and results, and follow all appropriate and current guidelines relative to human subject protection.

13. Ethical considerations in medical practice preclude the psychiatric evaluation of any adult charged with criminal acts prior to access to, or availability of, legal counsel. The only exception is the rendering of care to the person for the sole purpose of medical treatment.

14. Sexual involvement between a faculty member or supervisor and a trainee or student, in those situations in which an abuse of power can occur, often takes advantage of inequalities in the working relationship and may be unethical because: (a) any treatment of a patient being supervised may be deleteriously affected; (b) it may damage the trust relationship between teacher and student; and (c) teachers are important professional role models for their trainees and affect their trainees' future professional behavior.

Section 5

A physician shall continue to study, apply, and advance scientific knowledge, make relevant information available to patients, colleagues, and the public, obtain consultation, and use the talents of other health professionals when indicated.

1. Psychiatrists are responsible for their own continuing education and should be mindful of the fact that theirs must be a lifetime of learning.

2. In the practice of his/her specialty, the psychiatrist consults, associates, collaborates, or integrates his/her work with that of many professionals, including psychologists, psychometricians, social workers, alcoholism counselors, marriage counselors, public health nurses, etc. Furthermore, the nature of modern psychiatric practice extends his/her contacts to such people as teachers, juvenile and adult probation officers, attorneys, welfare workers, agency volunteers, and neighborhood aides. In referring patients for treatment, counseling, or rehabilitation to any of these practitioners, the psychiatrist should ensure that the allied professional or paraprofessional with whom he/she is dealing is a recognized member of his/her own discipline and is competent to carry out the therapeutic task required. The psychiatrist should have the same attitude toward members of the medical profession to whom he/she refers patients. Whenever he/she has reason to doubt the training, skill, or ethical qualifications of the allied professional, the psychiatrist should not refer cases to him/her.

3. When the psychiatrist assumes a collaborative or supervisory role with another mental health worker, he/she must expend sufficient time to assure that proper care is given. It is contrary to the interests of the patient and to patient care if he/she allows himself/herself to be used as a figurehead.

4. In relationships between psychiatrists and practicing licensed psychologists, the physician should not delegate to the psychologist or, in fact, to any nonmedical person any matter requiring the exercise of professional medical judgment.

5. The psychiatrist should agree to the request of a patient for consultation or to such a request from the family of an incompetent or minor patient. The psychiatrist may suggest possible consultants, but the patient or family should be given free choice of the consultant. If the psychiatrist disapproves of the professional qualifications of the consultant or if there is a difference of opinion that the primary therapist cannot resolve, he/she may, after suitable notice, withdraw from the case. If this disagreement occurs within an institution or agency framework, the difference should be resolved by the mediation or

arbitration of higher professional authority within the institution or agency.

Section 6

A physician shall, in the provision of appropriate patient care, except in emergencies, be free to choose whom to serve, with whom to associate, and the environment in which to provide medical services.

1. Physicians generally agree that the doctor-patient relationship is such a vital factor in effective treatment of the patient that preservation of optimal conditions for development of a sound working relationship between a doctor and his/her patient should take precedence over all other considerations. Professional courtesy may lead to poor psychiatric care for physicians and their families because of embarrassment over the lack of a complete give-and-take contract.
2. An ethical psychiatrist may refuse to provide psychiatric treatment to a person who, in the psychiatrist's opinion, cannot be diagnosed as having a mental illness amenable to psychiatric treatment.

Section 7

A physician shall recognize a responsibility to participate in activities contributing to an improved community.

1. Psychiatrists should foster the cooperation of those legitimately concerned with the medical, psychological, social, and legal aspects of mental health and illness. Psychiatrists are encouraged to serve society by advising and consulting with the executive, legislative, and judiciary branches of the government. A psychiatrist should clarify whether he/she speaks as an individual or as a representative of an organization. Furthermore, psychiatrists should avoid cloaking their public statements with the authority of the profession (e.g., "Psychiatrists know that . . .")

2. Psychiatrists may interpret and share with the public their expertise in the various psychosocial issues that may affect mental health and illness. Psychiatrists should always be mindful of their separate roles as dedicated citizens and as experts in psychological medicine.

3. On occasion psychiatrists are asked for an opinion about an individual who is in the light of public attention, or who has disclosed information about himself/herself through public media. It is unethical for a psychiatrist to offer a professional opinion unless he/she has conducted an examination and has been granted proper authorization for such a statement.

4. The psychiatrist may permit his/her certification to be used for the involuntary treatment of any person only following his/her personal examination of that person. To do so, he/she must find that the person, because of metal illness, cannot form a judgment as to what is in his/her own best interests and that, without such treatment, substantial impairment is likely to occur to the person or others.

GAP COMMITTEES AND MEMBERSHIP

COMMITTEE ON ADOLESCENCE
Warren J. Gadpaille, Denver, CO, Chairperson
Hector R. Bird, New York, NY
Ian A. Canino, New York, NY
Michael G. Kalogerakis, New York, NY
Paulina F. Kernberg, New York, NY
Clarice J. Kestenbaum, New York, NY
Richard C. Marohn, Chicago, IL
Silvio J. Onesti, Jr., Belmont, MA

COMMITTEE ON AGING
Gene D. Cohen, Washington, D.C. Chairperson
Eric D. Caine, Rochester, NY
Charles M. Gaitz, Houston, TX
Ira R. Katz, Philadelphia, PA
Andrew F. Leuchter, Los Angeles, CA
Gabe J. Maletta, Minneapolis, MN
Robert J. Nathan, Philadelphia, PA
George H. Pollock, Chicago, IL
Kenneth M. Sakauye, New Orleans, LA
Charles A. Shamoian, Larchmont, NY
F. Conyers Thompson, Jr., Atlanta, GA

COMMITTEE ON ALCOHOLISM AND THE ADDICTIONS
Joseph Westermeyer, Minneapolis, MN, Chairperson
Margaret H. Bean-Bayog, Lexington, MA
Susan J. Blumenthal, Washington, DC
Richard J. Frances, Newark, NJ
Marc Galanter, New York, NY
Edward J. Khantzian, Haverhill, MA
Earl A. Loomis, Jr., Augusta, GA
Sheldon I. Miller, Newark, NJ
Robert B. Millman, New York, NY
Steven M. Mirin, Westwood, MA
Edgar P. Nace, Dallas, TX
Norman L. Paul, Lexington, MA
Peter Steinglass, Washington, DC
John S. Tamerin, Greenwich, CT

COMMITTEE ON CHILD PSYCHIATRY
Peter E. Tanguay, Los Angeles, CA, Chairperson
James M. Bell, Canaan, NY
Harlow Donald Dunton, New York, NY
Joseph Fischhoff, Detroit, MI
Joseph M. Green, Madison, WI
John F. McDermott, Jr., Honolulu, HI
David A. Mrazek, Denver, CO
Cynthia R. Pfeffer, White Plains, NY
John Schowalter, New Haven, CT
Theodore Shapiro, New York, NY
Leonore Terr, San Francisco, CA

COMMITTEE ON COLLEGE STUDENTS
Earle Silber, Chevy Chase, MD, Chairperson
Robert L. Arnstein, Hamden, CT
Varda Backus, La Jolla, CA
Harrison P. Eddy, New York, NY
Myron B. Liptzin, Chapel Hill, NC

Malkah Tolpin Notman, Brookline, MA
Gloria C. Onque, Pittsburgh, PA
Elizabeth Aub Reid, Cambridge, MA
Tom G. Stauffer, White Plains, NY

COMMITTEE ON CULTURAL PSYCHIATRY
Ezra Griffith, New Haven, CT, Chairperson
Edward Foulks, New Orleans, LA
Pedro Ruiz, Houston, TX
Ronald Wintrob, Providence, RI
Joe Yamamoto, Los Angeles, CA

COMMITTEE ON THE FAMILY
Herta A. Guttman, Montreal, PQ Chairperson
W. Robert Beavers, Dallas, TX
Ellen M. Berman, Merrion, PA
Lee Combrinck-Graham, Evanston, IL
Ira D. Glick, New York, NY
Frederick Gottlieb, Los Angeles, CA
Henry U. Grunebaum, Cambridge, MA
Ann L. Price, Hartford, CT
Lyman C. Wynne, Rochester, NY

COMMITTEE ON GOVERNMENTAL AGENCIES
Roger Peele, Washington, DC, Chairperson
Mark Blotcky, Dallas, TX
James P. Cattell, San Diego, CA
Thomas L. Clannon, San Francisco, CA
Naomi Heller, Washington, DC
John P.D. Shemo, Charlottesville, VA
William W. Van Stone, Palo Alto, CA

COMMITTEE ON HANDICAPS
William H. Sack, Portland, OR, Chairperson
Norman R. Bernstein, Cambridge, MA
Meyer S. Gunther, Wilmette, IL
Betty J. Pfefferbaum, Houston, TX
William A. Sonis, Philadelphia, PA
Margaret L. Stuber, Los Angeles, CA
George Tarjan, Los Angeles, CA
Thomas G. Webster, Washington, DC
Henry H. Work, Bethesda, MD

COMMITTEE ON HUMAN SEXUALITY
Bertram H. Schaffner, New York, NY, Chairperson
Paul L. Adams, Galveston, TX
Johanna A. Hoffman, Scottsdale, AZ
Joan A. Lang, Galveston, TX
Stuart E. Nichols, New York, NY
Harris B. Peck, New Rochelle, NY
John P. Spiegel, Waltham, MA
Terry S. Stein, East Lansing, MI

COMMITTEE ON INTERNATIONAL RELATIONS
Vamik D. Volkan, Charlottesville, VA, Chairperson
Robert M. Dorn, El Macero, CA
John S. Kafka, Washington, DC
Otto F. Kernberg, White Plains, NY
John E. Mack, Chestnut Hill, MA
Peter A. Olsson, Houston, TX
Rita R. Rogers, Palos Verdes Estates, CA
Stephen B. Shanfield, San Antonio, TX

COMMITTEE ON MENTAL HEALTH SERVICES
Jose Maria Santiago, Tucson, AZ, Chairperson
Mary Jane England, Roseland, NJ
Robert O. Friedel, Richmond, VA
John M. Hamilton, Columbia, MD
W. Walter Menninger, Topeka, KS
Steven S. Sharfstein, Baltimore, MD
Herzl R. Spiro, Milwaukee, WI
William L. Webb, Jr., Hartford, CT
George F. Wilson, Somerville, NJ
Jack A. Wolford, Pittsburgh, PA

COMMITTEE ON PLANNING AND MARKETING
Robert W. Gibson, Towson, MD, Chairperson

Allan Beigel, Tucson, AZ
Robert J. Campbell, New York, NY
Doyle I. Carson, Dallas, TX
Paul J. Fink, Philadelphia, PA
Robert S. Garber, Longboat Key, FL
Richard K. Goodstein, Belle Mead, NJ
Harvey L. Ruben, New Haven, CT
Melvin Sabshin, Washington, DC
Michael R. Zales, Quechee, VT

Committee on Preventive Psychiatry
Naomi Rae-Grant, London, Ont., Chairperson
Viola W. Bernard, New York, NY
Stephen Fleck, New Haven, CT
Brian J. McConville, Cincinnati, OH
David R. Offord, Hamilton, Ont.
Morton M. Silverman, Chicago, IL
Warren T. Vaughan, Jr., Portola Valley, CA
Ann Marie Wolf-Schatz, Conshohocken, PA

Committee on Psychiatry and the Community
Kenneth Minkoff, Woburn, MA, Chairperson
C. Knight Aldrich, Charlottesville, VA
David G. Greenfield, Guilford, CT
H. Richard Lamb, Los Angeles, CA
John C. Nemiah, Hanover, NH
Rebecca L. Potter, Tucson, AZ
Alexander S. Rogawski, Los Angeles, CA
John J. Schwab, Louisville, KY
John A. Talbott, Baltimore, MD
Charles B. Wilkinson, Kansas City, MO

Committee on Psychiatry and Law
Jonas R. Rappeport, Baltimore, MD, Chairperson
Renee L. Binder, San Francisco, CA
John Donnelly, Hartford, CT
Carl P. Malmquist, Minneapolis, MN
Herbert C. Modlin, Topeka, KS
Phillip J. Resnick, Cleveland, OH
Loren H. Roth, Pittsburgh, PA
Joseph Satten, San Francisco, CA
William D. Weitzel, Lexington, KY
Howard V. Zonana, New Haven, CT

Committee on Psychiatry and Religion
Richard C. Lewis, New Haven, CT, Chairperson
Abigail R. Ostow, Belmont, MA
Sally K. Severino, White Plains, NY
Clyde R. Snyder, Fayetteville, NC

Committee on Psychiatry in Industry
Barrie S. Greiff, Newton, MA, Chairperson
Peter L. Brill, Radnor, PA
Duane Q. Hagen, St. Louis, MO
R. Edward Huffman, Asheville, NC
David E. Morrison, Palatine, IL
David B. Robbins, Chappaqua, NY
Jay B. Rohrlich, New York, NY
Clarence J. Rowe, St. Paul, MN
Jeffrey L. Speller, Cambridge, MA

Committee on Psychopathology
David A. Adler, Boston, MA, Chairperson
Jeffrey Berlant, Summit, NJ
John P. Docherty, Nashua, NH
Robert A. Dorwart, Cambridge, MA
Robert E. Drake, Hanover, NH
James M. Ellison, Watertown, MA
Howard H. Goldman, Potomac, MD
Anthony F. Lehman, Baltimore, MD
Kathleen A. Pajer, Pittsburgh, PA
Samuel G. Siris, Glen Oaks, NY

Committee on Public Education
Steven E. Katz, New York, NY, Chairperson
Jack W. Bonner, III, Asheville, NC

Jeffrey L. Geller, Worchester, MA
Keith H. Johansen, Dallas, TX
Elise K. Richman, Scarsdale, NY
Boris G. Rifkin, Branford, CT
Andrew E. Slaby, Summit, NJ
Robert A. Solow, Los Angeles, CA
Calvin R. Sumner, Buckhannon, WV

COMMITTEE ON RESEARCH
Robert Cancro, New York, NY, Chairperson
Jack A. Grebb, New York, NY
John H. Greist, Madison, WI
Jerry M. Lewis, Dallas, TX
John G. Looney, Durham, NC
Sidney Malitz, New York, NY
Zebulon Taintor, New York, NY

COMMITTEE ON SOCIAL ISSUES
Ian E. Alger, New York, NY, Chairperson
William R. Beardslee, Waban, MA
Judith H. Gold, Halifax, N.S.
Roderic Gorney, Los Angeles, CA
Martha J. Kirkpatrick, Los Angeles, CA
Perry Ottenberg, Philadelphia, PA
Kendon W. Smith, Pearl River, NY

COMMITTEE ON THERAPEUTIC CARE
Donald W. Hammersley, Washington, DC, Chairperson
Bernard Bandler, Cambridge, MA
Thomas E. Curtis, Chapel Hill, NC
Donald C. Fidler, Morgantown, WV
William B. Hunter, III, Albuquerque, NM
Roberto L. Jimenez, San Antonio, TX
Milton Kramer, Cincinnati, OH
Theodore Nadelson, Jamaica Plain, MA
William W. Richards, Anchorage, AK

COMMITTEE ON THERAPY
Allen D. Rosenblatt, La Jolla, CA, Chairperson
Gerald Alder, Boston, MA
Jules R. Bemporad, Boston, MA
Eugene B. Feigelson, Brooklyn, NY
Robert Michels, New York, NY
Andrew P. Morrison, Cambridge, MA
William C. Offenkrantz, Carefree, AZ

CONTRIBUTING MEMBERS
Gene Abroms, Ardmore, PA
Carlos C. Alden, Jr., Buffalo, NY
Kenneth Z. Altshuler, Dallas, TX
Francis F. Barnes, Washington, DC
Spencer Bayles, Houston, TX
C. Christian Beels, New York, NY
Elissa P. Benedek, Ann Arbor, MI
Sidney Berman, Washington, DC
H. Keith H. Brodie, Durham, NC
Charles M. Bryant, San Francisco, CA
Ewald W. Busse, Durham, NC
Robert N. Butler, New York, NY
Eugene M. Caffey, Jr., Bowie, MD
Ian L.W. Clancey, Maitland, Ont.
Sanford I. Cohen, Coral Gables, FL
Paul E. Dietz, Newport Beach, CA
James S. Eaton, Jr., Washington, DC
Lloyd C. Elam, Nashville, TN
Stanley H. Eldred, Belmont, MA
Joseph T. English, New York, NY
Louis C. English, Pomona, NY
Sherman C. Feinstein, Highland Park, IL
Archie R. Foley, New York, NY
Sidney Furst, Bronx, NY
Henry J. Gault, Highland Park, IL
Alexander Gralnick, Port Chester, NY
Milton Greenblatt, Sylmar, CA
Lawrence F. Greenleigh, Los Angeles, CA
Stanley I. Greenspan, Bethesda, MD
Jon E. Gudeman, Milwaukee, WI
Stanley Hammons, Lexington, KY
William Hetznecker, Merion Station, PA
J. Cotter Hirschberg, Topeka, KS
Jay Katz, New Haven, CT
James A. Knight, New Orleans, LA
Othilda M. Krug, Cincinnati, OH
Judith Landau-Stanton, Rochester, NY

Alan I. Levenson, Tucson, AZ
Ruth W. Lidz, Woodbridge, CT
Orlando B. Lightfoot, Boston, MA
Norman L. Loux, Sellersville, PA
Albert J. Lubin, Woodside, CA
John A. MacLeod, Cincinnati, OH
Charles A. Malone, Barrington, RI
Peter A. Martin, Lake Orion, MI
Ake Mattsson, Charlottesville, VA
Alan A. McLean, Westport, CT
David Mendell, Houston, TX
Roy W. Menninger, Topeka, KS
Mary E. Mercer, Nyack, NY
Derek Miller Chicago, IL
Richard D. Morrill, Boston, MA
Joseph D. Noshpitz, Washington, DC
Mortimer Ostow, Bronx, NY
Bernard L. Pacella, New York, NY
Herbert Pardes, New York, NY
Marvin E. Perkins, Salem, VA
David N. Ratnavale, Bethesda, MD
Richard E. Renneker, West Los Angeles, CA
W. Donald Ross, Cincinnati, OH
Donald J. Scherl, Brooklyn, NY
Charles Shagrass, Philadelphia, PA
Miles F. Shore, Boston, MA
Albert J. Silverman, Ann Arbor, MI
Benson R. Snyder, Cambridge, MA
David A. Soskis, Bala Cynwyd, PA
Jeanne Spurlock, Washington, DC
Brandt F. Steele, Denver, CO
Alan A. Stone, Cambridge, MA
Perry C. Talkington, Dallas, TX
Bryce Templeton, Philadelphia, PA
Prescott W. Thompson, Portland, OR
John A. Turner, San Francisco, CA
Gene L. Usdin, New Orleans, LA
Kenneth N. Vogtsberger, San Antonio, TX
Andrew S. Watson, Ann Arbor, MI
Joseph B. Wheelwright, Kentfield, CA
Robert L. Williams, Houston, TX
Paul Tyler Wilson, Bethesda, MD
Sherwyn M. Woods, Los Angeles, CA
Kent A. Zimmerman, Menlo Park, CA

LIFE MEMBERS

C. Knight Aldrich, Charlottesville, VA
Bernard Bandler, Cambridge, MA
Walter E. Barton, Hartland, VT
Viola W. Bernard, New York, NY
Murray Bowen, Chevy Chase, MD
Henry W. Brosin, Tucson, AZ
John Donnelly, Hartford, CT
Merrill T. Eaton, Omaha, NE
O. Spurgeon English, Narberth, PA
Stephen Fleck, New Haven, CT
Jerome Frank, Baltimore, MD
Robert S. Garber, Longboat Key, FL
Robert I. Gibson, Towson, MD
Paul E. Huston, Iowa City, IA
Margaret M. Lawrence, Pomona, NY
Jerry M. Lewis, Dallas, TX
Harold I. Lief, Philadelphia, PA
Judd Marmor, Los Angeles, CA
Karl A. Menninger, Topeka, KS
Herbert C. Modlin, Topeka, KS
John C. Nemiah, Hanover, NH
Alexander S. Rogawski, Los Angeles, CA
Mabel Ross, Sun City, AZ
Julius Schreiber, Washington, DC
Robert E. Switzer, Dunn Loring, VA
George Tarjan, Los Angeles, CA
Jack A. Wolford, Pittsburgh, PA
Henry H. Work, Bethesda, MD

BOARD OF DIRECTORS

OFFICERS

President
Carolyn B. Robinowitz
Deputy Medical Director
American Psychiatric Association
1400 K Street, N.W.
Washington, DC 20005

President-Elect
Allan Beigel
30 Camino Español
Tucson, AZ 85716

Secretary
Doyle I. Carson
Timberlawn Psychiatric Hospital
P.O. Box 11288
Dallas, TX 75223

Treasurer
Charles B. Wilkinson
2055 Holmes
Kansas City, MO 64108

Board Members
Judith Gold
Harvey L. Ruben
Pedro Ruiz
John Schowalter

Past Presidents

*William C. Menninger	1946-51
Jack R. Ewalt	1951-53
Walter E. Barton	1953-55
*Sol W. Ginsburg	1955-57
*Dana L. Farnsworth	1957-59
*Marion E. Kenworthy	1959-61
Henry W. Brosin	1961-63
*Leo H. Bartemeier	1963-65
Robert S. Garber	1965-67
Herbert C. Modlin	1967-69
John Donnelly	1969-71
George Tarjan	1971-73
Judd Marmor	1973-75
John C. Nemiah	1975-77
Jack A. Wolford	1977-79
Robert W. Gibson	1979-81
*Jack Weinberg	1981-82
Henry H. Work	1982-85
Michael R. Zales	1985-87
Jerry M. Lewis	1987-89

PUBLICATIONS BOARD

Chairman
Alexander S. Rogawski
11665 W. Olympic Blvd. #302
Los Angeles, CA 90064

C. Knight Aldrich
Robert L. Arnstein
Judith H. Gold
Milton Kramer
W. Walter Menninger
Robert A. Solow

Consultant
John C. Nemiah

Ex-Officio
Alan Beigel
Carolyn B. Robinowitz

CONTRIBUTORS
Abbott Laboratories
American Charitable Fund
Dr. and Mrs. Richard Aron
Mr. Robert C. Baker
Maurice Falk Medical Fund
Mrs. Carol Gold
Grove Foundation, Inc.
Miss Gayle Groves
Ittleson Foundation, Inc.
Mr. Barry Jacobson
Mrs. Allan H. Kalmus
Marion E. Kenworthy—Sarah H. Swift Foundation, Inc.
Mr. Larry Korman
McNeil Pharmaceutical
Phillips Foundation
Sandoz, Inc.
Smith Kline Beckman Corporation
Tappanz Foundation, Inc.
The Upjohn Company
van American Foundation, Inc.
Wyeth Laboratories
Mr. and Mrs. William A. Zales

---
*deceased

GAP Reports Published by Brunner/Mazel, Inc.

A Casebook in Psychiatric Ethics, Report #129

Crisis of Adolescence—Teenage Pregnancy: Impact on Adolescent Development, Report #118

A Family Affair: Helping Families Cope with Mental Illness: A Guide for the Professions, Report #119

The Family, the Patient, and the Psychiatric Hospital: Toward a New Model, Report #117

How Old is Old Enough? The Ages of Rights and Responsibilities, Report #126

Interactive Fit: A Guide to Nonpsychotic Chronic Patients, Report #121

The Mental Health Professional and the Legal System, Report #131

Psychiatric Prevention and the Family Life Cycle, Report #127

The Psychiatric Treatment of Alzheimer's Disease, Report #125

Psychiatry and the Mental Health Professionals: New Roles for Changing Times, Report #122

Psychotherapy with College Students, Report #130

Research and the Complex Causality of the Schizophrenias, Report #116

Speaking Out for Psychiatry: A Handbook for Involvement with the Mass Media, Report #124

Suicide and Ethnicity in the United States, Report #128

Teaching Psychotherapy in Contemporary Psychiatric Residency Training, Report #120

Us and Them: The Psychology of Ethnonationalism, Report #123

For ordering information
and a complete listing of available reports

Brunner/Mazel, Inc.
19 Union Square West, New York, NY 10003
212-924-3344